Immunology
A Foundation Text

Basiro Davey

JOHN WILEY & SONS
Chichester · New York · Brisbane · Toronto · Singapore

Copyright © 1989 The Open University

Reprinted in January 1992 by John Wiley & Sons Ltd,
Baffins Lane, Chichester,
West Sussex PO19 1UD, England

First published 1989 by Open University Press

Other Wiley Editorial Offices

John Wiley & Sons. Inc., 605 Third Avenue,
New York, NT 10158-0012, USA

Jacaranda Wiley Ltd, G.P.O. Box 859, Brisbane,
Queensland 4001, Australia

John Wiley & Sons (Canada) Ltd, 22 Worcester Road,
Rexdale, Ontario M9W 1L1, Canada

John Wiley & Sons (SEA) Pte Ltd, 37 Jalan Pemimpin #05-04,
Block B, Union Industrial Building, Singapore 2057

This text is based on a course book for the Open University's
S325 course 'Biochemistry and Cell Biology' and is reproduced
with the permission of the Open University and the approval of
the course team. The author gratefully acknowledges the valued
contribution of academic colleagues who commented extensively
on earlier drafts of all or part of this book—in particular,
Anna Furth, Colin Walker and Sarah Bullock from the Department
of Biology at the Open University; Professor Norman Staines from
the Department of Immunology at King's College, University of
London; and Dr David Catty from the Department of Immunology,
The University of Birmingham. The editor, Julia Powell, the
graphic artist, Pam Owen, and the designer, Sian Lewis, have
contributed greatly to the book's educational value.

British Library Cataloguing in Publication Data
Davey, Basiro
  Immunology.
  1. Immunology
  I. Title
  574.2'9
ISBN 0 471 93212 4

Printed and bound in Great Britain by Dotesios Ltd, Trowbridge

CONTENTS

1 IMMUNITY TO INFECTION 5
  1.1 The impact of infectious disease 5
  1.2 The immune response 6
  1.2.1 Innate and adaptive immunity 6
  1.2.2 The potential of the immune response 10
  Summary of Chapter 1 10

2 INNATE IMMUNITY 11
  2.1 Physical and chemical barriers to infection 11
  2.2 Leukocytes 12
  2.2.1 Phagocytic white cells 14
  2.2.2 Cytotoxic white cells 15
  2.2.3 Inflammatory white cells 16
  2.3 Extracellular chemical defences 17
  2.3.1 Lysozyme 17
  2.3.2 Interferons 17
  2.3.3 Acute phase proteins 17
  2.3.4 Complement 17
  2.4 The acute inflammatory reaction 18
  Summary of Chapter 2 18

3 THE CELLS OF ADAPTIVE IMMUNITY 20
  3.1 Small lymphocytes 20
  3.1.1 Antigen specificity and clonal selection 20
  3.1.2 Clonal expansion and immunological memory 22
  3.1.3 Two families of small lymphocytes 22
  3.2 B cells and their functions 25
  3.2.1 Antigen recognition by B cells 25
  3.2.2 B cell activation 26
  3.2.3 The antibody response 27
  3.2.4 The action of secreted antibodies 28
  3.3 T cells and their functions 30
  3.3.1 T cell subsets 30
  3.3.2 The T cell antigen receptor and the major histocompatibility complex 31
  3.3.3 The function of MHC restriction 32
  3.3.4 Antigen processing and antigen presentation 33
  3.3.5 Cytokines and lymphokines 33
  3.4 T cell and B cell traffic through the body 37
  Summary of Chapter 3 39

4 THE MOLECULES OF ADAPTIVE IMMUNITY 40
  4.1. Molecules involved in antigen recognition 40
  4.1.1 A little history 40
  4.2 The antibody molecule 41
  4.2.1 Constant and variable regions 43
  4.2.2 The antigen binding site 44
  4.2.3 Antibody classes and their functions 48
  4.2.4 Antibodies are also antigens! 52

4.3 The immunoglobulin genes 52
  4.3.1 The generation of antibody diversity 53
  4.3.2 Immunoglobulin class switching 58
  4.4 The major histocompatibility complex 59
  4.4.1 Class I MHC molecules 60
  4.4.2 Class II MHC molecules 61
  4.4.3 The *MHC* genes 62
  4.5 The T cell antigen receptor 65
  4.5.1 The structure of the receptor 65
  4.5.2 The *TcR* genes 66
  4.5.3 Interaction with antigen and MHC 66
  4.6 The immunoglobulin supergene family 67
  Summary of Chapter 4 68

5 COLLABORATION AND ESCAPE 70
  5.1 Collaboration between innate and adaptive immunity 70
  5.1.1 Division of labour in the immune response 71
  5.2 Escape strategies 72
  5.2.1 Bacterial escape strategies 73
  5.2.2 Viral escape strategies 74
  5.2.3 Parasite escape strategies 74
  Summary of Chapter 5 75

6 ANTIGENS 76
  6.1 General features of antigens 76
  6.1.1 Size 76
  6.1.2 Structure 76
  6.1.3 'Foreignness' 78
  6.1.4 Charged and hydrophobic residues 78
  6.1.5 Flexibility 79
  6.2. Antigen–antibody interactions 79
  6.2.1 Affinity measurement 79
  6.2.2 Avidity 81
  6.2.3 Cross-reacting antigens 82
  6.3 B cell and T cell epitopes 84
  6.4 Allogeneic and zenogeneic antigens 85
  6.4.1 Blood group antigens 86
  6.4.2 Tissue-specific antigens 87
  6.4.3 Differentiation and embryonic antigens 88
  Summary of Chapter 6 88

7 APPLICATIONS OF ANTIGEN RECOGNITION 89
  7.1 Producing the antibodies 90
  7.1.1 Polyclonal antiserum production 90
  7.1.2 Monoclonal antibody production 92
  7.2 Antigen purification by immunoaffinity chromatography 94
  7.3 Precipitation of soluble antigens 95
  7.3.1 Immunodiffusion methods 96
  7.3.2 Immunoelectrophoresis methods 97

7.4	Agglutination of cell-bound antigens	98
7.5	Immunolabelling methods	99
7.5.1	Radioimmunoassays	101
7.5.2	Enzyme-linked assays	102
7.5.3	Immunoblotting	104
7.5.4	Immunohistochemistry	106
7.5.5	Leukocyte assays using labelled antibodies	106
7.6	Rosettes and plaques	107
7.7	Diagnostic and therapeutic uses of antibodies *in vivo*	108
	Summary of Chapter 7	110

8 MATURATION OF THE ADAPTIVE RESPONSE — 111

8.1	Immune competence in embryos and new-born mammals	111
8.2	B cell maturation	112
8.3	T cell maturation	114
8.3.1	The acquisition of self-MHC restriction	115
8.3.2	Generation of T cell antigen receptors	117
8.4	Immunological tolerance	118
8.4.1	The induction of self-tolerance	118
8.4.2	The artificial induction of tolerance in adult life	120
8.4.3	The breakdown of self-tolerance	121
	Summary of Chapter 8	122

9 REGULATION OF THE IMMUNE RESPONSE — 123

9.1	Regulation by antigen and antibody concentration	123
9.2	Regulation by receptor density	124
9.3	Regulation by immune cell circuits	125
9.3.1	Idiotype network regulation	126
9.4	Genetic control of immune responsiveness	128
9.5	Regulation by neuroendocrine mechanisms	130
	Summary of Chapter 9	131

10 DISORDERS OF IMMUNITY — 132

10.1	Immunopathology	132
10.2	Congenital immune deficiency	133
10.3	Induced immunosuppression	133
10.3.1	Ionising radiation and immunosuppressive drugs	133
10.3.2	Parasite-induced immunosuppression	134
10.3.3	Human immunodeficiency virus (HIV)	134
10.4	Cancers: immune deficiency or immune hyperactivity?	136
10.5	Genetic contribution to immune hyperactivity disorder	138
10.6	Hypersensitivity reactions	140
10.6.1	Type I: immediate hypersensitivity	140
10.6.2	Type II: antibody-dependent cytotoxic hypersensitivity	141
10.6.3	Type III: immune complex-mediated hypersensitivity	142
10.6.4	Type IV: delayed or cell-mediated hypersensitivity	142
10.7	Autoimmune diseases	145
	Summary of Chapter 10	147

SELF ASSESSMENT QUESTIONS (SAQs)	149
ANSWERS TO SAQs	153
OPTIONAL FURTHER READING	159
INDEX	160
ACKNOWLEDGEMENTS	168

CHAPTER 1
IMMUNITY TO INFECTION

Immunology is the branch of natural science concerned with the study of immune systems in animals throughout the animal kingdom. Immune systems have evolved to protect animals against infection by harmful microbes and parasites. They range from simple biochemical and cellular defence mechanisms in invertebrates such as sponges and worms, to the very complex networks of immune cells and molecules found in mammals and birds.

This Book aims to give you a basic understanding of immune mechanisms in mammals, with particular emphasis on human immunology and its relationship to health and disease. Immunology is a rapidly advancing area of research that has stimulated public interest in recent years as a result of progress in vaccine development and organ transplantation, and recognition of the devastating effects of immune system breakdown following infection with the virus that can lead to AIDS. Immunology overlaps with the biological disciplines of biochemistry, cell biology, genetics, physiology, microbiology and parasitology; it relies on methods and concepts derived from these disciplines and, in turn, contributes to them. In this first Chapter we aim to stimulate your interest in immunology and give you an overview of the terrain that is covered in subsequent Chapters.

1.1 The impact of infectious disease

Animals and plants, from the simplest to the most complex in organisation, are susceptible to harm from a vast range of infectious *microbes* and multicellular *parasites*. Microbes that cause disease are termed *pathogens* to distinguish them from harmless or beneficial ones, and they include certain bacteria, viruses, protozoa and fungi. Some multicellular parasites (such as ticks and lice) live on the surfaces of their hosts, with irritating consequences, but those parasites that infest the internal organs can be a far more serious threat to health. An animal that is infected with a pathogen or parasite is described as the **host** for that infectious organism. In humans, pathogens and parasites cause ill health, ranging from the mildly inconveniencing symptoms of the common cold to acute and sometimes rapidly fatal infections, such as cholera and influenza, or the chronic debilitating illnesses that characterise many parasitic diseases, such as malaria, sleeping sickness and bilharzia.

Although infectious diseases now account for less than two per cent of human mortality in modern industrialised countries such as the UK, non-fatal episodes of ill health due to infections are still considerable, accounting for more GP consultations than any other category of illness. In many Third World countries, where pathogens and parasites cause 70–80 per cent of deaths, tens of millions of people die from infectious diseases annually, and children under five are especially susceptible. In a single year, as many as 20 million children in Asia, Africa and Latin America may die from diarrhoeal infections alone. Worldwide, about a billion people are infested with parasitic worms and flukes, and more than 100 million suffer from malaria.

What reasons occur to you to explain the striking differences in ill health caused by pathogens and parasites in different parts of the world?

In Third World countries, poor sanitation and contaminated water and food supplies are the root cause of the spread of infection. Their effects are exacerbated by malnutrition and existing infections, which reduce the body's ability to resist disease. Vaccination programmes for preventable infections, such as measles and tuberculosis, are often patchy and inadequately funded, and effective vaccines do not yet exist for several important Third World diseases including malaria and cholera.

In modern industrialised countries, where the population is well nourished, supplied with clean water and food, and protected by public health measures, such as vaccination and sewage disposal, people expect to be free from the ravages of unchecked fatal infections. But the spread of AIDS (*Acquired Immune Deficiency Syndrome*) in the western world in the 1980s has undermined that expectation and focused attention on the importance of the immune system in protecting us from infectious disease.

AIDS was first recognised when apparently healthy young adults in Europe and the USA rapidly succumbed to a range of normally innocuous infections, for which there were no medical remedies. People with AIDS suffer particularly from pneumonias caused by an unusual fungus, diarrhoeas caused by several strains of bacteria, and a cancer of the blood vessels for which a virus may be the underlying cause. Greatly increased susceptibility to these 'opportunistic' infections has been shown to be the result of an attack by a previously unknown virus, called *Human Immunodeficiency Virus* (HIV), on the body's immune system. Infection with HIV can lead to the suppression of the normal biochemical and cellular mechanisms of the immune response, leaving the infected person defenceless against other pathogens, which he or she would normally eliminate without difficulty. In Third World populations that are already debilitated by malnutrition, malaria and other infections, the effects of HIV on the immune system are having even more devastating consequences than in developed countries. However, the serious threat to world health posed by HIV infection is still dwarfed by the threat of other infectious and parasitic diseases.

1.2   The immune response

Immune systems throughout the animal kingdom respond to the presence of infectious organisms in the tissues of the host animal by directing a damaging **immune response** against the intruders. The cells and molecules that make up the immune response collaborate through a finely balanced network of interactions. This enables them to *detect* microbes, parasites or their toxic products in the body; *communicate* information to other parts of the network; and *recruit* a coordinated, multi-pronged attack, which may destroy the infecting organism, or at least limit its damaging effects. If the immune response is successful at eliminating the pathogen or parasite, then internal controls exist to *suppress* it. The immune response also shows a developmental sequence during the maturation of the organism to adulthood. For example, it is less effective in new-born mammals than it is in adults, and effectiveness may decline in old age (see Chapter 8).

1.2.1.   Innate and adaptive immunity

Immune mechanisms in different kinds of animal vary enormously in their complexity, but it has been traditional in immunology to divide these mechanisms into two groups. The mechanisms of the immune response found in invertebrates and some 'lower' vertebrates, such as reptiles and cartilaginous fish, are collectively termed **innate immunity**. The term *innate* immunity (or *natural* immunity in some texts) implies that these immune mechanisms are 'inborn' in all animals, since members of very different phyla, from the most primitive to the most complex, have some form of innate immunity. 'Higher' vertebrates—mammals, birds, some amphibians and bony fish—have, in addition, a more sophisticated set of mechanisms at their disposal, known collectively as **adaptive immunity**. The term *adaptive* refers to the ability of these immune mechanisms (unlike those of innate immunity) to change in characteristic ways following an infection. Figure 1.1 summarises the development of innate and adaptive immunity in immune systems among invertebrate and vertebrate phyla.

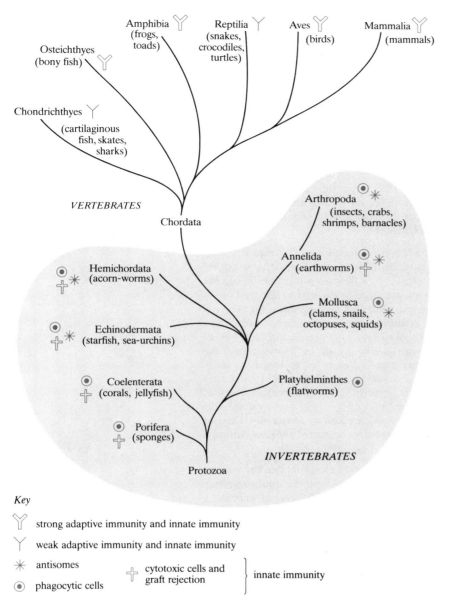

Key

Y strong adaptive immunity and innate immunity

Y weak adaptive immunity and innate immunity

⁎ antisomes

⊙ phagocytic cells

⊹ cytotoxic cells and graft rejection

} innate immunity

FIGURE 1.1 The development of complexity in the immune systems of invertebrate and vertebrate phyla. The terms in the key are explained in the text. Note that the vertebrates have both adaptive *and* innate immunity.

The distinction between innate and adaptive immunity has certain educational advantages in that it categorises a very complex set of immune mechanisms into two more readily understood groups. But this distinction also has an important disadvantage in that it has tended to obscure the high level of interdependence between the two types of immunity in higher vertebrates. The most modern immunology texts focus on the *interactions* between innate and adaptive immunity, which are discussed in Chapters 2, 3 and 5 of this Book.

The mechanisms of innate immunity always involve specialised **phagocytic** cells, or **phagocytes**. All vertebrates and multicellular invertebrates have these roving cells, which engulf foreign particles, debris or microbes in much the same way as an amoeba engulfing particles of food. The ingested foreign material is destroyed by potent intracellular enzymes and chemicals. This process is called **phagocytosis** ('cell eating') and is an important feature of the immune response throughout the animal kingdom. Several invertebrate phyla and all vertebrates also have **cytotoxic cells**, which kill infectious organisms by secreting toxic molecules on to them or by puncturing their surface membranes. Invertebrates of some phyla can use these mechanisms to reject tissue grafts, even from closely related species; sponges, corals, starfish and annelid worms have all been shown to be capable of **graft rejection**.

Moreover, some of the cellular and biochemical mechanisms involved in primitive immune responses resemble the most specialised immune mechanisms found in higher vertebrates. Earthworms and invertebrates from several other phyla can manufacture proteins (called *antisomes*). These bind to foreign molecules that have been introduced experimentally, and may aid the elimination of such molecules by phagocytosis. Antisomes have functional similarities to (and may be evolutionary precursors of) the *antibody* molecules that higher vertebrates manufacture as part of the adaptive immune response. The mechanisms of innate immunity in mammals will be discussed in detail in Chapter 2.

Innate immunity relies on cells that have *general* receptors for foreign material. Although pathogens and parasites have distinctive molecular structures, the receptors on innate immune cells do not bind to them in a selective or specific manner. Thus, all innate immune cells are activated to respond to the presence of any foreign material in much the same way. For this reason, innate immunity is sometimes referred to as *non-specific* immunity. In contrast, higher vertebrates have evolved immune systems that are able to detect the presence of each type of infectious organism very specifically by recognising ligands in the structure of the pathogen or parasite. These ligands are small clusters of molecules (usually polypeptides, glycoproteins or glycolipids) that occur in particular molecular conformations in the structure of infectious organisms or the macromolecules that they secrete. These molecular conformations do not normally occur on the cells and macromolecules of the host's own body and are known as **epitopes**. Cells or macromolecules that have epitopes in their structure are termed **antigens**. Antigens are the subject of Chapter 6.

Each cell involved in adaptive immunity has specialised receptors that can bind to epitopes with a complementary shape. This enables the adaptive immune response to be highly *specific*. It can be directed against a particular infectious agent because the pathogen or parasite has certain characteristic epitopes in its structure that 'fit' the receptors of adaptive immune cells. Although the epitope represents only a small portion of the structure of the infectious organism, the interaction of the epitope with the complementary receptor on an adaptive immune cell triggers an immune response that can destroy the intruder.

One group of adaptive immune cells is know as **B lymphocytes** or B cells. They *secrete* their receptors in large amounts, and these secreted receptor molecules are called **antibodies**. Another group of adaptive immune cells is known as **T lymphocytes** or T cells. These cells are involved in *regulating* the immune response, in inducing *inflammation* around infection sites and, directly, in *cytotoxicity* ('cell killing'). The activity of B lymphocytes and T lymphocytes is described in detail in Chapter 3, and the structure of their receptors is the subject of Chapter 4.

Another property that distinguishes adaptive from innate immunity is **immunological memory**. In this context, 'memory' does not imply any similarity with the mechanisms of memory storage in the brain. However, the term is useful in describing changes in the adaptive immune response following the experience of an infection. The innate immune response to a particular infectious agent is more or less the same no matter how many exposures to that agent the host organism has experienced. By contrast, the adaptive immune response becomes very much more effective when a particular type of pathogen or parasite is encountered for a second time. Thus, it is convenient to think of the adaptive immune system as retaining some sort of immunological memory of any infectious agent that it has encountered before.

When a pathogen infects a higher vertebrate for the first time, a **primary adaptive response** occurs, which is relatively slow to commence and lasts a few weeks at most. If the *same* pathogen is introduced a second time, a greatly enhanced **secondary response** occurs, which starts sooner, lasts longer and displays greater levels of activity than the primary response. The enhanced secondary response to a pathogen (and occasionally to a parasite) may be sufficiently effective to prevent subsequent infections from causing any symptoms, in which case the host animal is said to be **immune** to that pathogen. But the host does not display heightened immunity to infection by other *unrelated* pathogens that it has never encountered before, because each type of pathogen is recognised by its characteristic epitopes and responded to individually, in a specific way. The immunological memory applies only to those epitopes that have been encountered before. The mechanisms underlying immunological memory are described in Chapter 3.

☐ From what you know about adaptive immunity, what do you think a vaccine might contain, and what is the rationale for vaccination?

■ Vaccines contain antigens found in the structure of, or secreted by, a particular pathogen. They may contain killed whole organisms, harmless organisms that have similar antigens to the pathogenic species, inactivated toxic molecules that the pathogen secretes, or—increasingly—synthetic antigens constructed by protein biochemists. The rationale for vaccination is that exposing a person for the first time to the antigens in the vaccine will elicit a primary adaptive response and an immunological memory of those antigens without the person becoming ill. If the antigens are encountered subsequently on a live pathogen, the enhanced secondary response will be effective enough to eliminate it with, at worst, only mild symptoms of the disease.

Thus, in contrast to innate immunity, adaptive immunity is *specific* and, through the aquisition of immunological memory, the adaptive immune system can recognise any infectious organism it has encountered before. However, despite the lack of specificity and immunological memory, innate immunity is *not* inferior or ineffective: it contributes vital components to the defensive armoury of higher vertebrates, and is the main defence against infection in more primitive animals. As more research is carried out on invertebrate immunology, examples of weakly adaptive responses are being discovered. Some species of annelid worms have shown a small improvement in the speed at which they reject the second skin graft from another species of worm, indicating that their immune system has retained some sort of memory of the previous graft from that species.

Another reason for caution in ascribing a superior role to adaptive immunity in higher vertebrates is that the adaptive response is not always well controlled or entirely successful. The adaptive immune response in humans is generally more effective against bacteria and viruses than it is against parasites, with which it maintains at best an uneasy truce. In some circumstances, the adaptive immune response itself may cause significant harm to tissues surrounding the site of infection, and there are a number of important diseases in which the immune response is directed against inappropriate targets, including normal body cells and tissues. A critical feature of an effective immune response is its ability to distinguish accurately between the cells and macromolecules of the organism that is generating the response, and the cells and macromolecules of the pathogen or parasite against which the response is to be mounted. The adaptive immune system normally exhibits **self-tolerance**, that is, the *inability* to mount a damaging immune response against the body's own cells and macromolecules unless they have been altered by infection with pathogens or parasites, or by exposure to some chemicals or drugs. However, self-tolerance can break down, with very serious consequences. We return to disorders of the immune system in the final Chapter of this Book. The regulation of the adaptive immune response is the subject of Chapter 9.

1.2.2 The potential of the immune response

Before concluding this introduction to immunology, it is worth emphasising the immense potential of the immune response in protecting us from infection. The range of antigens that can be detected by the adaptive immune systems of higher vertebrates is enormous. Research into the receptors on adaptive immune cells has shown that there are at least 100 million receptor shapes; therefore the cells have the capacity to recognise (bind to) at least 100 million different epitopes. This receptor capacity enables the adaptive immune system to recognise a huge number of different antigens, for example, the cells or secreted products of pathogens and parasites, the cells of other individuals of the same species (as demonstrated by graft rejection), and even newly-synthesised molecules that can never have figured in our evolutionary history.

☐ Can you suggest why the adaptive immune system has evolved the potential to recognise such a wide range of antigens?

■ This huge potential enables the immune system to respond to new strains of infectious organism that may arise by mutation. New strains might have epitopes in their structure that have never occurred in nature before. The 'library' of receptors in the immune system is large enough to include some that could (by chance) bind to epitopes of the future.

The vast diversity of antigens that the adaptive immune system can recognise, coupled with the specificity of its response, has made immunology a subject of enormous interest to biological and medical science and to industry. The immune response exquisitely demonstrates certain fundamental biological principles. As you will see later, it illustrates the dependence of cellular and biochemical *function* on the *structure* of molecules on the surface of, and secreted by, cells of the immune system; and it offers many striking examples of the importance of *communication*, via receptor–ligand interactions, between cells involved in targeting and regulating the immune response. In addition, molecules produced by the immune system —particularly antibodies—have important *applications* as industrial, medical and research tools, as you will see in Chapter 7.

Summary of Chapter 1

1   Infectious diseases caused by pathogens and parasites account for millions of deaths annually, particularly in Third World countries. Prevention of infectious diseases depends on provision of uncontaminated water and food; safe sewage disposal; adequate nutrition and hygiene; vaccination and treatment (where effective interventions exist); and the normal functioning of the immune system.

2   AIDS has focused attention on the importance of the immune system in protecting people from infectious disease even in modern industrialised countries. Vaccination and organ transplantation have also aroused public interest in immunology.

3   Invertebrate and 'lower' vertebrate immune systems exhibit *innate immunity*, a non-specific, generally non-adaptive immune response, which can neither distinguish between different infectious organisms nor become more effective on subsequent exposure. Phagocytic and cytotoxic cells are important elements of innate immunity.

4   'Higher' vertebrates exhibit innate immunity plus *adaptive immunity*, a specific, adaptive immune response, which distinguishes very accurately between different infectious organisms and mounts a more effective response on second or subsequent exposure. Adaptive immunity displays specificity and immunological memory, and relies on B and T lymphocytes (B and T cells).

5   The cells involved in adaptive immunity have receptors that bind to *epitopes* (foreign molecular conformations) in the structure of pathogens and parasites. A cell or macromolecule that has epitopes in its structure is called an *antigen*; these include synthetic molecules and the cells of other individuals of the same species.

6   Animals are normally *self-tolerant*, that is, the immune system does not attack the animal's own body cells. However, the immune response is sometimes directed inappropriately against body cells or may over-react to foreign material, causing significant damage to normal tissues.

7   The huge diversity of receptors for antigens within the adaptive immune system gives the potential for specific responses to occur against new antigens formed by mutation. Receptor diversity has found many applications in biochemistry, industry and medicine.

Now attempt SAQs 1–3, which relate to this Chapter.

CHAPTER 2
INNATE IMMUNITY

This Chapter briefly reviews the cells and molecules that play a major role in innate (i.e. non-specific, non-adaptive) immunity in higher vertebrates, with particular emphasis on humans. We aim to demonstrate the vital role of these mechanisms in maintaining health, and to show that innate immunity forms the foundation on which adaptive immunity rests.

2.1   Physical and chemical barriers to infection

Skin on the external surfaces of the body, and the mucous membranes that line the gut, respiratory and genital tracts are important **physical and chemical barriers to infection**. Most pathogens cannot penetrate intact skin, and bacterial survival on the surface of human skin is inhibited by the low pH of sweat and secretions from sebaceous glands. Other mechanisms for preventing the entry of pathogens into the tissues include acid in gastric secretions; the anti-bacterial enzyme *lysozyme* in breast milk, tears, nasal secretions and saliva; harmless bacteria living in the gut and genital tract, which compete for survival against infectious bacteria and fungi; anti-bacterial proteins and zinc in semen; the layer of protective mucus secreted by mucous membranes; and mechanical movements of cilia in the bronchial tubes, aided by coughing and sneezing reflexes (Figure 2.1).

All these physical and chemical barriers to infection may be considered to be part of the innate immune system, since they are non-specific and do not become more effective after exposure to a particular pathogen. However, barriers can be breached. The skin can be damaged by cuts, grazes and burns, which allow pathogens and parasites to enter, and some bacteria can break down the barriers with enzymes. Infectious organisms can also get into the gut in food and water, or into the respiratory tract on air currents or microscopic droplets of water, or they may be introduced by insect or other animal vectors (for example, mosquitos transmit the malarial parasite in their saliva while taking a blood meal). Most of the chemical barriers are only weakly effective against viruses, and various mechanisms have been evolved by infectious organisms to evade these barriers and gain entry to the body (as you will see in Chapter 5). Thus, a second line of defence is necessary, and this relies on several types of cell, collectively called *leukocytes*.

First line defence is physical/chemical barriers (as mentioned)

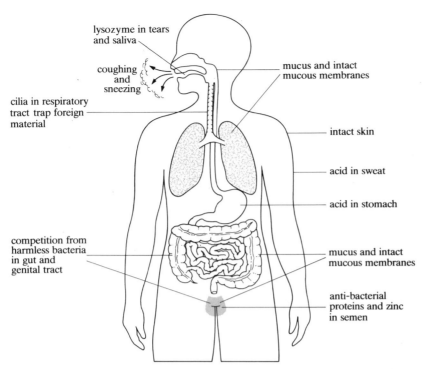

FIGURE 2.1 Summary of the main physical, chemical and mechanical barriers to infection entering the human body.

2.2 Leukocytes

Leukocytes (from the Greek *leukos*, meaning white) are often called *white blood cells*, but this term creates the incorrect impression that these cells are always to be found in the bloodstream. In fact, some leukocytes are never found in the vascular circulation, and those that do enter it spend only a very small proportion of their lifespan there. In this Book we will use either *leukocytes* or *white cells* when we need a collective term for the many different cell types that collaborate in an immune response.

Figure 2.2 shows the origin of all mammalian leukocytes, red cells and platelets to be a single pool of precursor cells, called ~~multipotent~~ **stem cells,** in the bone marrow, which differentiate to give several families or 'lineages' of cells. As few as 30 of these stem cells are sufficient to regenerate the entire white and red cell population of a mouse after the original cells have been destroyed by radiation. You will need to refer to Figure 2.2 a number of times during this Chapter as we describe some of the cell types shown, and we will refer to it again in Chapter 3.

The names given to the different types of leukocyte generally tell you something about their function, biochemistry or morphology. The **lymphoid cells** spend most of their lifespan in the *lymphoid system*, which consists of organs such as the lymph nodes, tonsils and spleen, connected by a network of lymphatic capillaries. We will describe the lymphoid system in more detail in the next Chapter because it is the major location of adaptive immune responses mediated by *small lymphocytes*.

The **granulocytes** all have numerous electron-dense structures in their cytoplasm, which stain in characteristic ways when treated with different histological dyes. Granulocytes that do not stain with either acidic or alkaline dyes are known as *neutrophils*, whereas *eosinophils* stain with acidic dyes (of which *eosin* is one), and

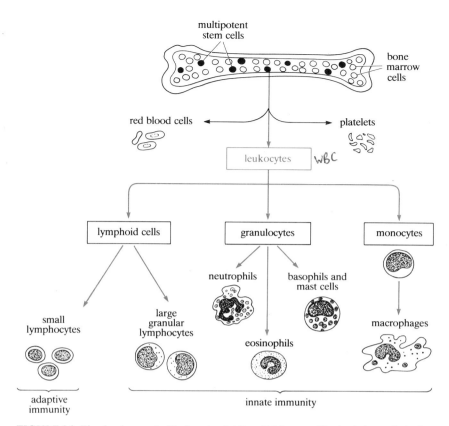

FIGURE 2.2 The development of leukocytes (white cells) from multipotent stem cells in the bone marrow of mammals. There are three main lineages of white cells: the *lymphoid cells*, the *granulocytes* and the *monocytes*. Adaptive immunity is mediated by the small lymphocytes and innate immunity by all the other types of white cell, but resistance to infection relies on many interactions between these two groups of cells.

basophils and *mast cells* stain with alkaline (basic) dyes. We will describe their functions in innate immunity in Sections 2.2.1 to 2.2.3, but first a word about terminology.

The darkly-staining structures that are so characteristic of granulocytes are always referred to in immunology texts as *granules*. This term suggests a solid particle, like a grain of sand, which is exactly how these structures appeared to the early microscopists who named them. Closer examination under an electron microscope reveals that the granules are in fact membrane-bound 'packets', which contain numerous biologically active molecules, including enzymes and toxins. A more accurate biological term for these structures would be *vesicles*, since they resemble the vesicles that contain biologically active molecules in other cell types (e.g. vesicles of neurotransmitter substances in nerve cells). But, since immunologists always refer to white-cell vesicles as 'granules', we will follow the tradition in this Book.

The third main lineage of white cells is the **monocytes**, which migrate out of the blood capillaries and into tissues and organs all around the body, where they differentiate into *macrophages*. Macrophage literally means 'big eater', from which you can deduce that these cells are phagocytic.

Innate immunity relies on the activity of certain lymphoid cells, together with the various types of granulocytes and monocytes. The activity of all these cells can be divided into three categories: *engulfing* foreign material (phagocytosis), *killing* infectious organisms by damaging the cell membrane (cytotoxicity), and generating *inflammation* around the site of an infection.

2.2.1 Phagocytic white cells

Two types of white cell are mainly responsible for destroying pathogens by phagocytosis: these are the *neutrophils* and the *macrophages*. (Eosinophils are also capable of phagocytosis but this is not their main function.) **Neutrophils** are the most numerous of the white cells found in the bloodstream, contributing between 50 and 70 per cent of the total 'white count'. They are easy to recognise in microscope slides because of their multi-lobed nucleus (Plate 2.1a), which has given rise to the long form of their name, *polymorphonuclear* neutrophils. They live only a few days and do not divide once they have entered the bloodstream. **Macrophages** are the largest of the white cells and have a characteristic horseshoe or kidney-shaped nucleus (Plate 2.1b). Less than seven per cent of white cells circulating in the bloodstream are macrophages, but large numbers are found widely distributed throughout body tissues. Macrophages are highly mobile, long-lived cells that migrate through connective tissues by squeezing through the intercellular spaces. They are found close to the basement membrane that covers blood vessels, around the walls of the gut, in the genital tract and abundantly in the lungs, lymph nodes and spleen. Specialised macrophages (with specific names not mentioned here) are found in the liver, kidneys, brain and bones, and in the lymphoid system.

The different distribution of neutrophils and macrophages—neutrophils are found predominantly in the blood and macrophages in the tissues—ensures that whenever infectious organisms enter the body they are likely to encounter a phagocytic cell. **Phagocytosis** by neutrophils and by macrophages follow a similar course. The phagocytic cell must first adhere to the surface of the 'foreign body', which may be a pathogen, some cell debris or an inorganic particle such as grit. This raises two questions: how does the phagocyte recognise foreign material, and how does it adhere to its target?

Recognition of some types of bacteria involves receptors on the phagocyte cell membrane that bind to certain configurations of carbohydrate residues in the bacterial cell wall. In addition, specialised serum proteins bind to chemical groups in the cell walls of many types of pathogen and label them with a chemical 'tag' that identifies the pathogen as a target for phagocytosis. These chemical tags are known collectively as **opsonins**, and include *antibodies*, *acute phase proteins* and *complement*—all of which will be described later in this Chapter or in the next. Opsonins also have ligands in their structure, which bind to receptors in the membrane of the phagocytic cell. Thus, recognition and adherence may be effected by the same intermediary molecule (Figure 2.3). The coating of pathogens with proteins that promote phagocytosis is known as **opsonisation**, from the Greek *opson* meaning cooked meat, but a more memorable translation has been provided by the immunologist Ivan Roitt as 'made ready for the table'. The importance of opsonisation can be judged from the fact that it increases by many orders of magnitude the rate of elimination of encapsulated bacteria from the bloodstream.

Adherence of the phagocytic cell to a pathogen triggers a system of contractile actin–myosin filaments inside the phagocyte, which enables the cell to throw 'arms' (pseudopodia) of cytoplasm around the target and enclose it in membrane (Plate 2.2). The membrane surrounding the pathogen fuses with the membranes surrounding lysosomes in the phagocytic cell. Lysosomes are small intracellular packets of powerful degradative enzymes and toxic molecules, which are emptied on to the engulfed pathogen with destructive effect. Macrophages also have metabolic pathways that generate a burst of highly toxic derivatives of molecular oxygen inside the membrane enclosing the pathogen. These derivatives include hydrogen peroxide and various highly reactive free radicals (compounds with unpaired electrons) which, together with chloride ions, form a cocktail that is lethal to viruses as well as bacteria. These compounds are powerful *oxidising agents*; between them they can oxidise most of the chemical groups found in proteins, carbohydrates and lipids. Uncontrolled oxidation leads to the break-up of the pathogen because the lipids in its cell membrane are particularly sensitive to oxidation.

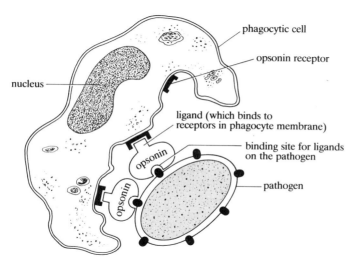

FIGURE 2.3 Opsonins form a bridge between phagocytic cells and their targets, aiding recognition and adherence, and increasing the rate of elimination of pathogens by phagocytosis. Important opsonins include antibodies, acute phase proteins and a component of complement. (*Note that in this diagram, as in many others that follow, the size of the surface receptors has been grossly exaggerated in relation to the size of the phagocyte; if they were drawn to the same scale the receptors would not be visible unless the cells were drawn at least as large as a dinner plate!*)

2.2.2   Cytotoxic white cells   (T-cells)

Cytotoxic cells are those that kill other cells directly by chemical means, without phagocytosis. Two types of cytotoxic activity are important in the innate immune response, one of which requires antibody molecules to be bound to the target, while the other does not. Cytotoxic activity that can occur in the *absence* of antibodies is carried out by two types of white cell: the *eosinophils* and some members of the *large granular lymphocyte* population.

Eosinophils form one to three per cent of white cells in the bloodstream. They stain intensely with acidic dyes, and have numerous intracellular 'granules' containing degradative enzymes and a cylindrical protein that can perforate cell membranes. Like macrophages, eosinophils can generate a burst of oxidising agents, but they direct this out of the cell on to the surface of the target. The adherence of eosinophils to targets that have been coated with opsonins (including antibody molecules) is greatly enhanced, and this improves their cytotoxic effect, but they are not *dependent* on opsonins. Their main role in innate immunity is to inflict damage on multicellular parasites, such as worms and flukes, that are too large to be phagocytosed.

Less than one per cent of white cells can carry out an *entirely* antibody-*independent* form of cytotoxicity, called **natural killer**, or **NK**, activity. NK activity is directed against a very restricted range of targets, primarily virus-infected body cells, but it is *non-specific* in that the same cell can kill a range of host cells infected with different viruses. White cells with this ability are all from the large granular lymphocyte population, and many immunology texts refer to them as **NK cells**, although it is not certain that they are a distinct type of cell with this as their sole function.

The receptor molecules in the surface membrane of white cells with NK activity bind to viral glycoproteins that appear on the surface of infected body cells as new virus particles are constructed. The adherent NK cell releases several biologically active proteins into the small space between its membrane and that of its target. One of these proteins, called **perforin**, is a cylindrical molecule that is inserted into the target-cell membrane, opening up a pore to the outside. Sodium ions flood into the target cell through many such pores, altering the osmotic balance so that water is drawn in by osmotic pressure. If enough pores are created, the osmotic pressure builds up to the point where the target cell bursts. NK activity can also be directed against certain malignant cells in tissue culture, but it is unlikely that this is significant in controlling human cancers. NK cells have no effect against 'free' virus particles, bacteria or parasites.

The white cells that carry out **antibody-dependent cell-mediated cytotoxicity** (**ADCC**) are also from the large granular lymphocyte population. Some texts refer to them as **K cells** (K for killer), but again it is not known if this is their sole function; they are not easy to distinguish functionally from cells with NK activity. As the term ADCC suggests, these cells can only kill targets that are coated with antibody molecules. The cytotoxic cell has receptors in its membrane for ligands that are part of the antibody molecule, so recognition of, and adherence to, the target are dependent on the presence of antibodies. The killing mechanisms are those already described for NK activity. Notice that although ADCC requires the presence of molecules synthesised by *adaptive* immune cells (i.e. antibodies), the cytotoxic cells involved in this type of killing are *non-specific* in their activity in that they can kill *any* cell that has *any* type of antibody bound to it. This is a good example of the interdependence of the mechanisms of innate and adaptive immunity.

2.2.3 Inflammatory white cells

Several types of white cell synthesise and secrete biologically active molecules that provoke an intense but **acute** (short-lived) **inflammatory reaction** around the site of an infection. Although macrophages and neutrophils contribute some of these molecules, two other cell types are particularly involved: the *basophils* and the *mast cells*.

Basophils circulate in the bloodstream whereas **mast cells** remain stationary in connective tissue, and are especially abundant in the respiratory tract. These two cell types are characterised by their densely granular cytoplasm, which stains intensely with alkaline dyes (Plate 2.3a). Certain stimuli cause these 'granules' to be expelled very rapidly from the cell (Plate 2.3b). An important mediator of degranulation is a type of antibody molecule, called IgE (see Chapter 4.2.3), which binds to the surface membrane of mast cells and basophils; the stimulus for degranulation is the binding of antigen to these surface-bound IgE molecules. The granules expelled from stimulated mast cells and basophils contain several biologically active compounds (including *histamine*), which cause local blood vessels to dilate and become leaky so that plasma and white cells flood out. The inflammatory reaction underlies the characteristic swelling, redness and heat that occur at the site of infection.

☐ What is the value of an inflammatory reaction in the protective immune response?

◼ The inrush of plasma brings a large number of phagocytic and cytotoxic cells to the infection site, together with molecules that aid their activity, for example, opsonins and antibodies.

Other biologically active molecules are also concentrated at the scene of an inflammatory reaction. These have a variety of functions including direct toxicity to pathogens and the immobilisation of white cells in the infection site. These *extracellular chemical defences* are an important component of innate immunity.

2.3 Extracellular chemical defences (cytokines?)

2.3.1 Lysozyme

One of the most important and abundant biochemical defences against unencapsu-lated strains of bacteria is the enzyme **lysozyme**. This is found in most external secretions, for example, sweat, tears and saliva (Figure 2.1), and in blood and intercellular fluid. It is secreted principally by macrophages. Lysozyme splits bonds between the amino sugars in *peptidoglycans*, the main components of bacterial cell walls. Peptidoglycans are *only* found in bacteria, so tissues throughout the body can safely be bathed in lysozyme. Breaking the bonds in peptidoglycans punctures the bacterial cell wall and kills the bacterium. However, many strains of bacteria have a capsule of protein and lipids *outside* the peptidoglycan layer, which acts as a barrier to lysozyme action. Opsonins can overcome this problem by 'labelling' the bacterium for phagocytosis.

2.3.2 Interferons

Another important group of molecules is the **interferons**, a family of proteins that are secreted by white cells during an immune response. Interferons have an inhibitory effect on further viral replication in neighbouring uninfected cells, possibly by triggering a chain of intracellular events that greatly reduce the rate of transcription of DNA into mRNA.

☐   How would this help to prevent further spread of the virus?

■   The reduction in mRNA transcription brings cell metabolism almost to a halt because no new proteins can be synthesised. If interferon-treated cells become infected by virus, the transcription of viral DNA into mRNA and translation into new virus proteins is greatly reduced. This creates a cordon of uninfect-able cells around the original site of infection, which limits further spread.

Interferons act *non-specifically* on host cells that are targets for any strain of virus, but they also have other important effects on cells involved in both innate and adaptive responses. For example, the activity of NK cells against virus-infected cells is greatly enhanced by exposure to interferons.

2.3.3 Acute phase proteins

A number of different proteins in the bloodstream increase in concentration very rapidly during an infection, reaching as much as 100 times their normal level. These molecules are known collectively as **acute phase proteins**, and their concen-tration can be monitored as an indicator of the progression or remission of an infection. Their main role is to act as opsonins by enhancing the rate of phagocytosis.

2.3.4 Complement

Complement is the collective term for a series of about 20 serum proteins that circulate in the body fluids in an inactive form. Several of these proteins are secreted by macrophages—yet another contribution to innate immunity by these versatile cells. When the first component of complement is activated, a complex **cascade reaction** is set in motion, in which the reaction products of each step in the sequence activate the next component in the cascade.

The first complement component can be activated by certain polysaccharides in the cell walls of some types of bacteria and parasites, by acute phase proteins bound to bacteria and to fungi, and by antibodies bound to foreign material. Thus, complement can be triggered both by certain infectious organisms and by the 'labelling' devices of opsonins and antibodies, and represents one of several important links between innate and adaptive immunity. The final products in the

Pierces membrane of pathogen — cause Lysis
— cause intracellular
contents of m/o cell
to leak.

complement cascade are known as the **membrane attack complex**, a cylindrical assembly of molecules that is inserted into the cell wall of the microbe or parasite, thus opening up a pore through which sodium ions, and then water, flood into the cell. The membrane attack complex bears a close structural similarity to *perforin* which, as you saw in Section 2.2.2, has a similar function in NK cytotoxicity.

Several of the intermediate complement components also have important functions. One of the most abundant components generated by the activated cascade is called C3b and is a potent opsonin. Two other components, known as C3a and C5a, stimulate the burst of oxidising agents in macrophages that proves so toxic to pathogens. They also contribute to the acute inflammatory reaction by triggering basophils and mast cells to degranulate. C5a is also a powerful **chemotactic factor**, that is, a chemical attractant for white cells, which causes them to migrate up the concentration gradient towards the factor's source. Other chemotactic factors are released when mast cells degranulate.

2.4   The acute inflammatory reaction

We conclude this Chapter by drawing together our discussion of the various white cells and molecules that contribute to innate immunity by summarising the **acute inflammatory reaction** (Figure 2.4). This reaction not only occurs at infection sites but also around cuts, burns and grazes to the skin, sealing them with an exudate of plasma, white cells and clotting factors that congeal into a protective scab.

As you study Figure 2.4, bear in mind that the reaction is accelerated by molecules secreted by the first cells to arrive; these molecules recruit more cells, which in turn release molecules that further enhance the reaction. For a time, *positive feedback* loops exist to ensure that the reaction, once triggered, proceeds very rapidly. As you would expect, inhibitory mechanisms also exist to damp down the reaction and prevent it from spreading, but if these mechanisms fail (as they sometimes do when the infection is persistent) then the inflammation can become chronic and serious damage results. An *allergic* inflammatory reaction can also be triggered in some people by non-infectious foreign material, such as pollen grains, house dust mites, animal fur and certain foods. We return to the subject of *allergies* and other inappropriate inflammatory reactions in the final Chapter of this Book.

In the next Chapter we turn to the more complex mechanisms of *adaptive* immunity, but before doing so it is worth emphasising that innate responses, including inflammatory reactions, begin within a few *hours* of infectious organisms entering the body. This is much faster than the responses of adaptive immunity, even when the pathogens have been encountered before. The mechanisms of innate immunity are the sole means of defence in the period of at least several days following an infection before a primary adaptive response can be detected.

Summary of Chapter 2

1   The first line of defence against infection is the physical barrier of skin and mucous membranes, aided by other physical, mechanical and chemical defences, such as mucus, the coughing reflex, and antibacterial and antiviral compounds.

2   The second line of defence is provided by many different types of *leukocyte*, or white cell, all of which (together with red blood cells and platelets) are derived from a single pool of *multipotent stem cells* in the bone marrow.

3   *Neutrophils* and *macrophages* are phagocytic white blood cells that engulf pathogens, foreign particles and cell debris, and destroy them with enzymes, acids and oxidising agents.

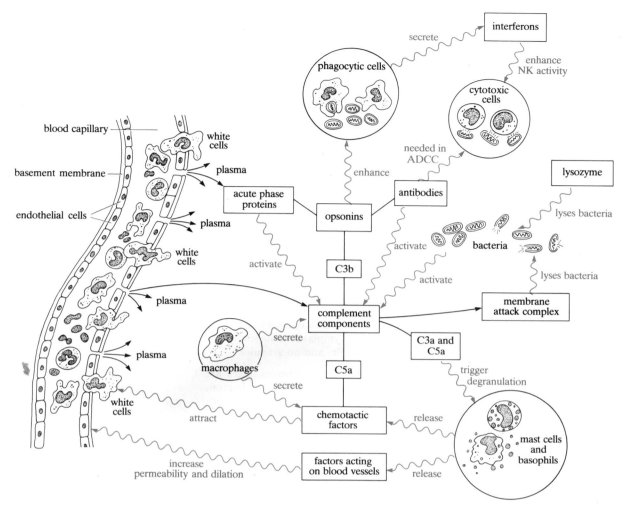

FIGURE 2.4 A summary of the mechanisms of innate immunity (aided by antibodies), which initiate and amplify an acute inflammatory reaction at the site of an infection. NK refers to natural killer activity; ADCC is antibody-dependent cell-mediated cytotoxicity; C3a, C3b and C5a are all intermediates in the complement cascade reaction. For further explanation, see text.

4 *Opsonisation* is the labelling of pathogen cell-membranes with a molecule (*opsonin*) that identifies the pathogen as a target for phagocytosis and aids adherence of the phagocyte to the pathogen; opsonisation greatly enhances the rate of pathogen elimination.

5 *Natural killer* (*NK*) cells are cytotoxic to virus-infected cells, and *eosinophils* primarily kill parasites. Both use pore-forming proteins and toxic molecules to damage the target cell membrane. *Antibody-dependent cell-mediated cytotoxicity* (*ADCC*) may also occur when cytotoxic cells bind to antibody-coated targets.

6 Extracellular chemical defences include *lysozyme*; *interferons* that inhibit virus replication and enhance NK activity; and *complement*, a system of serum proteins with many effects including opsonisation, triggering mast cell degranulation, chemotaxis, and pore formation in bacterial cell walls.

7 The *acute inflammatory reaction* involves capillary dilation, changes to capillary walls that allow white cells and plasma to flood out, and chemotaxis (chemical attraction of white cells). It is mediated by complement components, the contents of mast cell and basophil granules, and molecules secreted by macrophages.

Now attempt SAQs 4–7, which relate to this Chapter.

CHAPTER 3
THE CELLS OF ADAPTIVE IMMUNITY

This Chapter concentrates on the cells involved in adaptive immunity by describing the ways in which they recognise and respond to antigens in a healthy individual, and by explaining the cellular basis of *antigen specificity* and *immunological memory*. Immune cells interact with antigens and with each other by means of receptors and complementary ligands in their surface membranes. Thus, a description of immune *cells* inevitably draws us into describing the function of the most important cell-bound receptors and ligands: *antibodies*, the *T cell antigen receptor* and the molecules encoded by a set of genes called the *major histocompatibility complex* (or *MHC*). However, the detailed molecular structures and underlying genetic codes for these molecules are the subject of Chapter 4.

3.1 Small lymphocytes

The adaptive immune response rests on the activity of the white cells classified as **small lymphocytes**, aided by macrophages and other accessory cells. If you look back at Figure 2.2 you will see the developmental relationship of small lymphocytes to the other types of leukocyte. Small lymphocytes are recognisable under the light microscope because they have a very low ratio of cytoplasm to nucleus (Plate 3.1), and what little cytoplasm there is has few organelles and no granules.

Despite their homogeneous appearance under the light microscope, there are several types of small lymphocyte whose specialised functions in adaptive immunity are only revealed by their contact with *antigens*. The definition of an antigen is a cell or molecule that has ligands in its structure that are bound specifically by receptors in the membranes of small lymphocytes, or by the secreted form of B cell receptors (i.e. antibodies). These antigenic ligands are called *epitopes*. In the shorthand of immunology, a small lymphocyte *recognises* an antigen when the receptor molecule in the cell membrane binds to an epitope on the antigen (Figure 3.1). Notice that only a part of the receptor molecule has a complementary shape that binds to the epitope; this is called the **antigen binding site**. Thus, the interaction of a small area of an antigen (the epitope) and a small area of a lymphocyte receptor (the antigen binding site, or *paratope* in some texts) brings the antigen and the lymphocyte into close proximity.

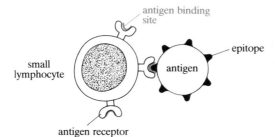

FIGURE 3.1 Antigen recognition by small lymphocytes requires the interaction of a ligand (here the epitope on an antigen) with the complementary binding site of an antigen receptor on the surface membrane of the lymphocyte.

3.1.1 Antigen specificity and clonal selection

You already know from Chapter 1 that a characteristic of the adaptive immune response is its ability to respond to each antigen independently of others. Thus, the epitopes on each antigen must be recognised by the adaptive immune system (i.e. the small lymphocytes) in a highly specific and selective manner. However, the small lymphocytes of an individual can, between them, recognise and distinguish at least 10^8 different epitopes. This implies that at least 10^8 different receptor molecules exist in the small lymphocyte population.

☐ In theory, this number could be achieved by each lymphocyte having receptor molecules for each of the millions of epitopes that it might encounter. What problems would this solution present?

■ There would not be space enough on the surface of each cell for adequate numbers of all these receptors, nor is there enough DNA in the nucleus to encode millions of different receptor proteins.

The solution to this problem is that each small lymphocyte has receptor molecules of unique structure and specificity that bind to just *one* epitope—or at most a few with very similar structures—so each cell requires the DNA necessary to encode only a single type of receptor. Each small lymphocyte is, in turn, a member of a **clone** of identical cells with identical receptors that bind to the same epitope (Figure 3.2a). But the population of small lymphocytes consists of *millions* of different clones, each clone with receptors for a particular epitope. Between them, the clones of small lymphocytes have the potential to recognise all the antigens that an individual might encounter in life—and many that have never been synthesised in nature. Thus, the ability of the immune system *as a whole* to recognise and respond to each antigen in a specific way rests on the fact that only those small lymphocytes with complementary receptors for particular epitopes will bind to antigens that carry those epitopes. This is referred to as **clonal selection** because, in effect, the antigen 'selects' the clone (or clones) that has receptors that will bind to it (Figure 3.2b). Lymphocytes from other clones cannot bind to it because their receptor molecules are the wrong shape.

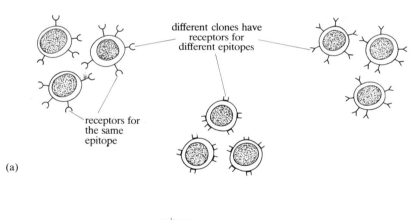

(a)

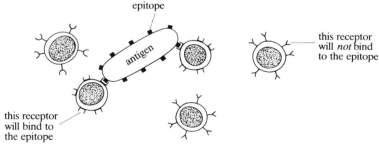

(b)

FIGURE 3.2 (a) Small lymphocytes are members of clones, each consisting initially of a few cells with receptors for the *same* epitope. Members of different clones have receptors for *different* epitopes. (b) Only the members of a clone with complementary receptors will bind to a particular epitope. Antigens therefore 'select' the clones with the appropriate receptors.

Note that most naturally occurring antigens have a number of different epitopes in their structure. Therefore, a bacterial cell, for example, might 'select' several clones, each with receptors for one of several epitopes in the bacterial cell wall or capsule.

At birth, each clone of lymphocytes consists of only a few cells since there is not space enough in the lymphoid system to pack in clones consisting of many thousands of cells. These original cells are referred to as **naive lymphocytes,** (or virgin lymphocytes) signifying that they are committed to recognise a particular epitope (i.e. they have the correct receptors) but have not yet encountered it. However, the few naive cells in each clone are not sufficient to mount an effective immune response, which normally utilises many thousands of lymphocytes with receptors for a particular antigen. The answer to this conundrum lies in the process of *clonal expansion,* which also underlies another characteristic feature of adaptive immunity— *immunological memory.*

3.1.2 Clonal expansion and immunological memory

When an antigen enters the body and 'selects' a particular lymphocyte (or perhaps several) by receptor–epitope binding, the original cells replicate several times. This process is known as **clonal expansion** (Figure 3.3).

Maturation and differentiation also take place during this expansion phase. Most of the new cells formed are *effector cells* of various kinds, which act to eliminate the antigen in ways that we will describe in a moment. When the antigen has been destroyed, the effector cells die, so each clone expands and then contracts as the need for an immune response wanes. But some of the new cells formed during clonal expansion differentiate into **memory cells**. The memory cells are lymphocytes with a long life that continue to circulate in the body after the original exposure to the antigen is over and the effector cells have died. They form an enlarged clone of lymphocytes committed to respond rapidly, by clonal expansion and differentiation into effector cells, if the same antigen is encountered again. Even without contact with antigen, memory cells generally replicate at intervals to replenish the pool of memory cells, so they may offer life-long protection against many antigens.

☐ How do clonal selection and clonal expansion explain the susceptibility of a person to (say) a particular strain of influenza virus when they encounter it for the first time, and their ability to shrug off the infection if they are exposed to the same virus at a later date?

■ At first exposure, the immune response has to start from the relatively small clones of naive lymphocytes with appropriate receptors for the viral epitopes. By the time clonal expansion has taken place and an effective *primary* immune response is underway, viral replication may have reached a level sufficient to produce the symptoms of influenza. After recovery, however, an expanded pool of memory cells with receptors for the epitopes of this virus persists. This pool forms the basis of a more rapid *secondary* response if the virus is encountered again, which may be effective enough to prevent symptoms from arising. Thus effective immunity is not evident to the 'infected' person.

Clonal selection by antigen and the consequent clonal expansion underlie the ability of the adaptive response to be directed very specifically against a particular antigen. The formation of memory cells accounts for the difference between the *primary* and the *secondary adaptive response* to an antigen, which we discussed in Chapter 1, and also explains the protective effect of vaccination.

3.1.3 Two families of small lymphocytes

We mentioned earlier that several types of lymphocyte exist, each type performing a specialised function in adaptive immunity. There are two main families: the **B lymphocytes** (or simply **B cells**), which mature after contact with antigen into

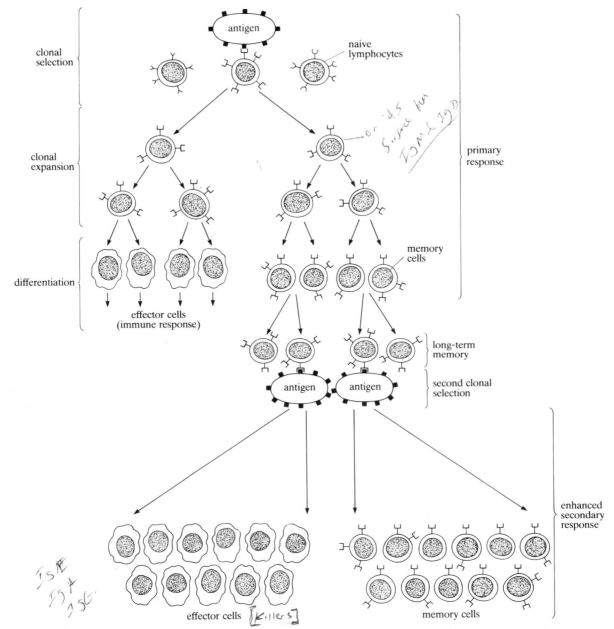

FIGURE 3.3 Clonal selection, clonal expansion and differentiation during the primary and secondary adaptive immune responses to an antigen. The expansion in cell numbers at each stage is several orders of magnitude greater than shown here. The effector cells have a life of only a few days, whereas the memory cells survive for months or even years.

antibody-secreting cells; and the **T lymphocytes** (or **T cells**), which regulate the immune response, are involved in prolonged inflammatory reactions, and kill infected body cells. In Sections 3.2 and 3.3 we describe each of these families in more detail; but bear in mind that they are both made up of clones of cells, each with receptors for a particular epitope, and each undergoing clonal selection, expansion and memory-cell formation when activated by the appropriate signals, including contact with a specific antigen.

The term 'B cell' originated because it was first discovered that antibody-secreting cells in birds matured in an organ unique to birds called the Bursa of Fabricius; if the Bursa is removed from newly hatched chicks then they are completely unable to synthesise antibodies. Thus, B cell originally stood for 'Bursa-dependent' cell. But, fortuitously, it was later discovered that B cells in mammals matured in the *bone marrow* (and to some extent in foetal liver), so B cell has come to mean 'bone marrow-dependent' cell (Figure 3.4).

By contrast, the precursors of T cells in all higher vertebrates leave the bone marrow in which the lymphoid cell lineage first develops from multipotent stem cells (Figure 2.2) and migrate to the thymus, an organ located behind and slightly above the heart. Differentiation into mature T cells occurs in the thymus, and T cell stands for 'thymus-dependent' cell (Figure 3.4).

There has been a tradition in immunology to think of the adaptive immune response in two parts, known as **humoral immunity** and **cell-mediated immunity**. *Humoral* immunity encompasses the molecules, secreted by small lymphocytes, that could be detected in the body fluids, and thus focuses primarily on antibodies and the B cells from which they are derived. *Cell-mediated* immunity refers to the direct actions of immune cells on each other, on cellular antigens, and on infected body cells, and thus focuses primarily on the actions of T cells. This distinction is being steadily eroded as it becomes ever clearer that B cells are more than simply antibody factories, and that T cells secrete numerous complex molecules, which are essential to antigen recognition and for co-ordinating the immune response.

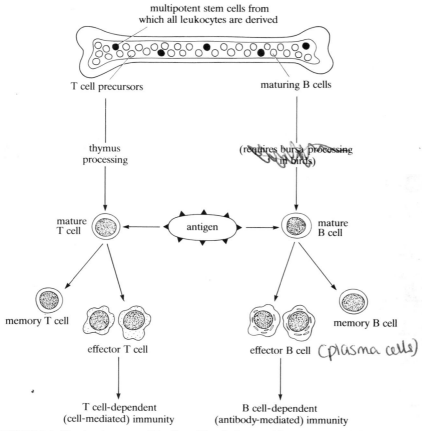

FIGURE 3.4. The development of T cells and B cells from multipotent stem cells in the bone marrow of mammals and birds. Traditionally, cell-mediated (T cell-dependent) and anti-body-mediated (B cell-dependent) immunity have been considered separately, but the *interdependence* of T cells and B cells has now been extensively demonstrated.

24

3.2 B cells and their functions

3.2.1 Antigen recognition by B cells

The antigen receptors on all B cells are known as **antibodies**. More accurately, these receptor molecules are described as **surface immunoglobulins**, or simply **sIg** (pronounced *ess-eye-gee* or *sig*), denoting that they are globular proteins in the surface membrane of an immune cell and have an immunological function. B cells are the only type of cell in the body to have surface immunoglobulins, so the presence of sIg on a cell membrane is a useful identifying **marker molecule for B cells**. (As you will see later, different identifying marker molecules can be found on T cells.) Each B cell has about 10^5 sIg molecules in its surface membrane.

B cells bind to an antigen via the binding sites in the sIg molecules, which interact with complementary epitopes on the antigen (Figure 3.5a). Antigen binding, together with certain activating signals from T cells, causes the original B cell to proliferate. The expanded clone differentiates into memory cells and **plasma cells** (the effectors). Plasma cells synthesise and secrete large amounts of virtually the same immunoglobulin molecules that the original B cell used as its surface receptor for antigen. (In fact, the secreted immunoglobulins lack the short hydrophobic section that acts as the anchor for the sIg molecule in the B cell membrane, but are otherwise identical to sIg molecules.) These secreted immunoglobulins are the *antibodies* that appear in the bloodstream and tissue fluids. We look at the detailed molecular structure of immunoglobulins in the next Chapter, but the general plan of a secreted immunoglobulin or antibody molecule is shown in Figure 3.5b.

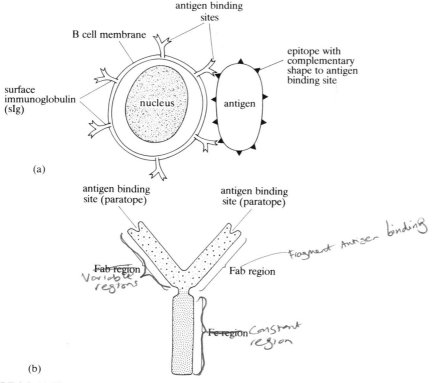

FIGURE 3.5 (a) The B cell's receptors for antigen consist of molecules of immunoglobulin embedded in the cell membrane with their antigen binding sites facing outwards. The size of the surface immunoglobulin molecules (or sIg) has been grossly exaggerated in this Figure. (b) Antibodies in the circulation are secreted immunoglobulin molecules, conventionally represented as a Y-shaped structure. There are two identical antigen binding sites (or paratopes) at the tips of the two Fab regions (Fab = *F*ragment *a*ntigen *b*inding). The single Fc region (Fc = *F*ragment *c*rystallisable) is so called because pure preparations of Fc regions readily crystallise.

The antibody molecule is Y-shaped and can be cleaved by enzymes into three parts: two identical **Fab regions** and a single **Fc region**. The terms for these parts were coined in the 1950s when it was discovered that each of the Fab regions could bind to the appropriate antigen (Fab stands for 'fragment antigen binding'), whereas the Fc region did not bind to the antigen but could be crystallised (Fc stands for 'fragment crystallisable'). Notice in Figure 3.5b that there are two identical binding sites (also referred to as *paratopes* in some texts) at the tips of the Fab regions. When the antibody molecule is anchored in the B cell membrane by a hydrophobic section of polypeptide attached to the Fc region, these binding sites face outwards.

The Fc region of the molecule has a relatively *constant* primary structure from one antibody molecule to the next, but the Fab regions *vary* greatly in their primary structure when antibody molecules secreted by different clones of plasma cells are compared. The primary structure of the Fab regions determines the higher-order structure of the binding site, and hence its shape and charge profile. This in turn determines which ligands will fit into the binding site. Thus the *antigen specificity* of each antibody molecule is a consequence of the higher-order structure of its Fab regions.

One final point about the B cell antigen receptor should be emphasised. Antibodies (and hence B cells) bind to 'native' antigens, i.e. intact antigenic macromolecules as they occur in life, either free in the body fluids or as part of the surface structure of an infectious organism. As you will see later in this Chapter, this is very different from what the T cells recognise as an antigen.

3.2.2   B cell activation

Antigen binding is an *essential* requirement for the activation of most B cells, and for a minority of B cells it is also a *sufficient* activating signal. However, most B cell clones require antigen binding plus additional signals from *T cells* before they can begin clonal expansion (Figure 3.6a). Antigens can therefore be classified as **T cell dependent** and **T cell independent**.

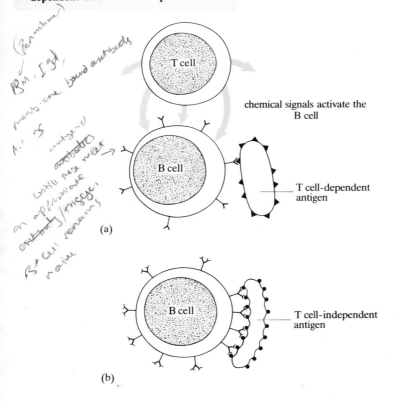

FIGURE 3.6 (a) Most B cells require antigen binding *and* chemical signals from a T cell before the B cell is activated to begin clonal expansion. Antigens that cannot activate a B cell without T cell help are termed T cell-dependent antigens. (b) A few antigens are T cell-*independent* and activate B cells in the absence of T cells. Some of these antigens are polymers with repeating unit structures, which activate the B cell by cross-linking a number of adjacent antigen receptors (sIg molecules).

26

The rest of this Book is concerned with those antigens that require T cell 'help' before B cell activation occurs, so we will refer briefly here to the antigens that can activate B cells independently. Some bacterial cell walls (e.g. those of *Streptococcus pneumoniae*, which causes pneumonia) contain antigenic polysaccharides, which have regularly spaced, repeating, unit structures and are able to *cross-link* several adjacent molecules of sIg on the surface of the B cell (Figure 3.6b). This cross-linking is sufficient to trigger the B cell to begin the phase of clonal expansion and differentiation into mature, antibody-secreting plasma cells. B cells may also be activated *regardless* of their antigen specificity by certain **polyclonal activators**. These include powerful *mitogens* (compounds that cause cells to undergo mitosis), some of which are also components of bacterial cell walls. Another polyclonal activator is the *Epstein-Barr virus*, which is involved in the causation of an immune-cell cancer (Burkitt's lymphoma). Relatively few T cell-independent antigens exist in life. Most antigens will not fully activate their matching B cell in the absence of molecular signals from T cells, even when many sIg molecules have bound to it. We will discuss the nature of these activating signals shortly, when we look at T cells in more detail.

Before moving on, note that many complex cellular processes are subsumed under the deceptively simple word *activation*. This word encompasses all the changes in cell metabolism and gene expression that enable the cell to divide, differentiate and become a factory for secreted antibodies.

3.2.3 The antibody response

Once B cell activation has taken place, plasma cells differentiate during clonal expansion, and synthesise and secrete large amounts of immunoglobulin, all of which has identical binding sites for one type of antigen. The rate of appearance of secreted antibodies in the circulation of a person who has encountered a particular antigen for the *first* time (i.e. the primary response) differs in characteristic ways from the rate of appearance of antibodies after a second encounter (i.e. the secondary response). This is illustrated in Figure 3.7.

☐ What are the principal differences shown in Figure 3.7 between the primary and secondary responses in terms of antibody secretion?

■ There are three differences. (a) There is a lag of about ten days before detectable levels of antibody appear in the serum after first exposure to the antigen, whereas the lag phase is only about three or four days in the secondary response. (b) Antibody concentration rises more rapidly and reaches much higher levels during the secondary response. (c) Antibody levels decline quite quickly during the primary response, and in this case are undetectable after about a month, whereas they persist for much longer after a secondary response (in fact, for months or even years).

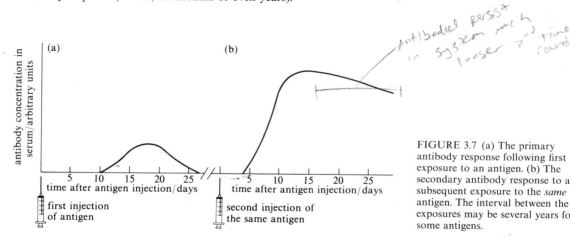

FIGURE 3.7 (a) The primary antibody response following first exposure to an antigen. (b) The secondary antibody response to a subsequent exposure to the *same* antigen. The interval between the two exposures may be several years for some antigens.

You should have no difficulty in explaining these phenomena in terms of clonal expansion of the appropriate B cells following the first exposure to the antigen, and the formation of memory B cells, which initiate the secondary response. However, remember that during the long lag phase before antibodies are formed during the primary response, the mechanisms of innate immunity are already mounting a strenuous defence against the antigen.

3.2.4   The action of secreted antibodies

When secreted antibodies become bound to their matching antigen, they *facilitate* its destruction in a number of ways but, contrary to popular belief, they are not directly toxic to the antigen. Antibodies exert most of their various effects by *enhancing* the mechanisms of innate immunity, as you will see from the following list, which describes their action and serves as a revision of Chapter 2. The effects of secreted antibodies are summarised in Figure 3.8.

1   Since antibody molecules have *two* binding sites for antigen, a single molecule of antibody can bind two molecules of antigen together, and many antibody molecules can bind many antigen molecules together to form a lattice. Large clumps of antigen are more easily phagocytosed by macrophages and polymorphs than are single molecules.

2   Bound antibodies *opsonise* antigens, i.e. label them as targets for phagocytosis and facilitate phagocyte adherence to the antigen. Phagocytes have receptors in their surface membranes that bind to ligands in the Fc region of antibody molecules. (By comparing part 2 of Figure 3.8 with Figure 2.3 you can see how antibodies act as opsonins.)

3   Bound antibodies also form a bridge between antigens and K cells, and between parasite cells and eosinophils, increasing the killing power of the cytotoxic cells. In addition, phagocytes can be transformed into cytotoxic cells by the antibody bridge if it connects them to a target that is too large to be engulfed (e.g. a parasite). Binding to the Fc part of the antibody stimulates the phagocyte to externalise its lysosomes, and so empty their toxic contents over the surface of the parasite. These mechanisms are collectively termed *antibody-dependent cell-mediated cytotoxicity*, or ADCC for short.

4   When bound to antigens, antibodies trigger the complement cascade. The sequence of intermediates is different from the sequence triggered by bacterial-wall polysaccharides and acute phase proteins (see Chapter 2) but the end-product —the membrane attack complex—and the lytic effect on bacterial cells are the same.

5   The activation of complement by bound antibodies also contributes to a local inflammatory response because C3a and C5a cause mast cell degranulation. In addition, a particular type of antibody (called immunoglobulin E) has the ability to bind to mast cells and cause degranulation when it, in turn, binds to antigen.

In the next Chapter you will see how the *structure* of the antibody molecule enables it to perform these varied *functions*.

☐   In all the cases described in the list, the antibody molecule has to be bound to its matching antigen before it can activate or enhance the innate effector mechanism. What is the value of this?

■   It ensures that 'free' antibodies in the circulation do not set off an inflammatory response, so that inflammatory responses don't occur indiscriminately; they can only do so in the immediate vicinity of the antigen.

Notice also that the antibodies themselves have no direct toxic or lytic effect on the antigen—they simply 'label' it as a target for phagocytic or cytotoxic cells, which are themselves unable to recognise antigens with the exquisite specificity that B cells and antibodies can achieve.

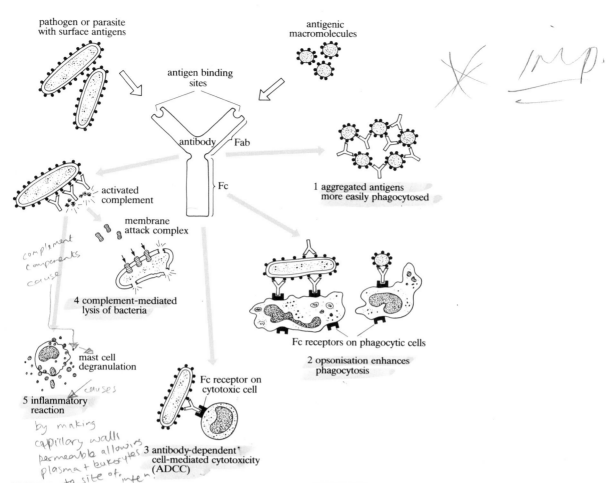

FIGURE 3.8 Summary of the ways in which secreted antibodies activate, focus and enhance the mechanisms of innate immunity. Numbers relate to more detailed descriptions of these processes in the text (Section 3.2.4).

Antibodies also have an effector function that is not dependent on innate immunity. It relies, instead, on the ability of bound antibodies to interfere with the biochemical structure of the antigen and hence to alter its activity. For example, the toxins secreted by some bacteria (such as *Corynebacterium diphtheriae*, which causes diphtheria) are also antigens; if the epitopes are in, or close to, the active site of the toxin, then antibody binding may interfere with the ability of the toxin to combine with its target molecule and hence to cause harm. Antibodies bound to epitopes that are distant from the active site of the toxin may still interfere with its toxic activity by inducing conformational changes in the toxin that alter its active site (this is called *allosteric* inhibition). Some virus particles may also be prevented from binding to their target cell by similar interference from bound antibodies. Attempts to develop a vaccine that will protect people from infection with human immunodeficiency virus (HIV) have included trying to elicit antibodies that interfere with the virus in this way.

However, antibody-mediated immune responses are most effective against free-living pathogens, parasites and antigenic macromolecules in the circulation; they do not easily reach the many types of pathogen, including viruses, that replicate and live inside the cells of their host. Our main defence against these intracellular pathogens is the T cells.

3.3. T cells and their functions

T cells have three main functions in adaptive immunity: to *kill* body cells that have become infected with pathogens and that are therefore inaccessible to antibodies; to maintain an *inflammatory response* at the site of a persistent infection (e.g. around a multicellular parasite); and to *regulate* many features of both the adaptive and innate immune responses.

3.3.1   T cell subsets

Not suprisingly, given the variety of functions that T cells perform, the T cell population is divided into several **subsets**, each with specialised functions (Figure 3.9). The killing function is carried out by **cytotoxic T cells** (T_c). These cells use toxic and pore-forming chemicals to kill the body's own cells, when they have become infected with intracellular pathogens, in much the same way as described earlier for NK cells. The regulatory functions are carried out by **helper T cells** (T_h), which synthesise and secrete a range of molecules with activating or enhancing effects on other cells involved in the immune response. **Suppressor T cells** (T_s) have the opposite effect—they prevent the activation of other immune cells, or cause them to reduce their activity or cease functioning altogether. The cells involved in prolonged inflammatory reactions are part of the helper T cell subset; they are sometimes referred to as a separate group (the *delayed-type hypersensitivity T cells*), but we include them with the helper T cells in this Book.

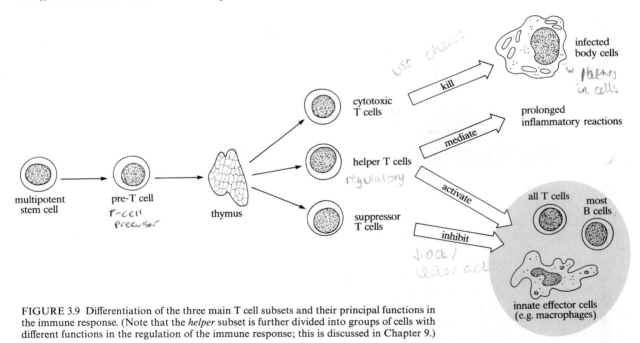

FIGURE 3.9 Differentiation of the three main T cell subsets and their principal functions in the immune response. (Note that the *helper* subset is further divided into groups of cells with different functions in the regulation of the immune response; this is discussed in Chapter 9.)

The cells in each of these subsets have characteristic *marker molecules* in their surface membranes that enable them to recognise each other (and which, incidentally, also allow their identification in the laboratory). All of these marker molecules are receptors for ligands on the surface of other cells or for ligands on secreted molecules, and they appear on the T cell surface at a certain stage of cell differentiation. Each of these molecules has been given an internationally agreed *CD number* (CD stands for cluster of differentiation; the term derives from the fact that these molecules are characteristic of a particular type of differentiated cell). The distribution of CD molecules on T cell subsets is shown in Table 3.1, together with the main marker molecules that distinguish other white cells involved in the immune response.

TABLE 3.1 Some of the major surface marker molecules that characterise human cells involved in the immune response

Cell type	Surface marker molecules
all T cells	CD2*, CD3, CD11
helper T cells	CD4
suppressor and cytotoxic T cells	CD8
all B cells	sIg; Epstein-Barr virus receptor**; Fc receptors (for the 'tail' region of antibodies)
macrophages, neutrophils, eosinophils, basophils and mast cells	complement component receptors and Fc receptors

* CD2 molecules are involved in cell-to-cell adhesion interactions, and coincidentally also bind to a surface molecule on the red blood cells of sheep; binding to sheep red cells is one way of identifying T cells *in vitro*.
** It is not known why B cells have a receptor for this virus.

3.3.2 The T cell antigen receptor and the major histocompatibility complex (MHC)

All T cells—whatever their subset—also carry receptor molecules, which are anchored in the surface membrane and have binding sites for a particular epitope. Like the B cells, each T cell can recognise and bind to a single type of epitope or, at most, a very few biochemical analogues of it. When an antigen enters the body it 'selects' T cells with complementary receptors. However, the **T cell antigen receptor** is not a molecule of antibody, although it has certain structural similarities to the immunoglobulins, as you will see in the next Chapter. It consists of a number of different polypeptides; some of these contain binding sites for a particular epitope, some have binding sites for ligands on other cells, and some are involved in signal transduction, i.e. transmitting the information to the T cell nucleus that antigen has been correctly bound. For now, it is enough to note that each T cell receptor 'recognises' its matching epitope with the same degree of precision that B cells achieve with surface immunoglobulin.

There is another fundamental contrast with B cells in the way in which T cells recognise antigen. This flows from their role in identifying body cells that are harbouring intracellular pathogens. Unlike sIg, which binds to antigen alone, the T cell antigen receptor binds simultaneously to antigen *and* a cluster of molecules that occur on the surface membrane of virtually all cells in the body (Figure 3.10). These molecules are the products of a cluster of genes known as the *major histocompatibility complex*, generally abbreviated to *MHC*. (Note that in this book we will follow the accepted convention of printing the names of *genes* in italics, and their products in upright type; thus, *MHC* genes encode MHC molecules.)

Although the **MHC molecules** of all humans are structurally closely related, there are significant differences in the structure of these molecules from one person to the next. This is because each gene in the complex is just one of a huge number of different *alleles* (i.e. different forms), and it is highly improbable that any two non-identical individuals will inherit the *same* set of alleles. Only identical twins inherit the same alleles and hence express the same MHC molecules on their body cells. We discuss the detailed structure of the MHC molecules and the genes that encode them in the next Chapter; for the moment you should note that they are divided into two groups, known as *class I* and *class II*. Each subset of T cells has receptors that bind to antigens only when the antigen is in association with a particular class of MHC molecule—a phenomenon known as **MHC restriction**. The T cell antigen receptor binds not only to the antigen but also to ligands in the MHC molecules (Figure 3.10). MHC molecules with broadly similar structures and functions have also been found on the cells of several species of rodents, rabbits and sheep, and it seems likely that they are distributed widely throughout the mammals.

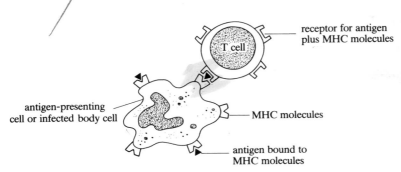

FIGURE 3.10 The T cell antigen receptor can only bind to the antigen when it is 'presented' to the T cell in association with 'self' major histocompatibility complex (MHC) molecules. This restricts T cells to recognising antigens *only* when they are on the surface of the host's own cells.

3.3.3 The function of MHC restriction

Class I MHC molecules are found on virtually every cell in the body of those mammalian species that have been investigated. If a cell is infected with an intracellular pathogen, such as a virus, fragments of antigenic glycoproteins from disintegrating pathogens, or from new pathogens under construction, appear in the surface membrane of the infected cell. These antigenic fragments tend to associate in the cell membrane with the class I MHC molecules. The antigen receptor on *cytotoxic* T cells is constructed so that it can only bind to the epitope of an antigen if the antigen is associated with class I MHC molecules—it cannot bind to antigen alone. Moreover, the MHC molecules must be *identical* to those on the T cell.

☐ What is the consequence of restricting cytotoxic T cells in this way?

■ Cytotoxic T cells only recognise antigens when they are on the surface of the body's *own* cells, and thus they are specially adapted to mount an immune response to pathogens that 'hide' inside the cells of their host. They ignore extracellular pathogens such as 'free-living' bacteria, or free virus particles, which are dealt with by the innate immune system and antibodies.

Class II MHC molecules are found primarily on *activated* leukocytes. One of the many consequences of activation by antigen and other signals is that the genes encoding the class II molecules in T cells, B cells, macrophages and some other leukocytes are transcribed and expressed at the cell surface. These molecules have an important role in regulating the immune response by placing restrictions on which immune cells can interact with each other. *Helper* T cells (and possibly suppressor T cells) can only bind to an antigen when it is associated with class II MHC molecules in the surface membrane of another activated leukocyte from the same individual. The antigen receptors of each helper T cell are restricted to binding with a specific foreign epitope in association with ligands in the class II

MHC molecules. Antigenic fragments can associate with class II molecules at the cell surface in much the same way as we have already described for class I. For example, antigenic fragments appear in the cell surface when phagocytes break down engulfed pathogens or antigenic macromolecules or when they become infected with intracellular pathogens. Moreover, B cells in contact with antigen can internalise it and then re-express it at the cell surface in association with class II molecules.

☐ What is the value of class II MHC restriction?

■ It restricts each helper T cell to interacting only with those leukocytes that have *also* recognised the antigen for which the T cell has receptors. Thus, MHC restriction focuses T cell 'help' on to precisely those immune cells that are required to mount an effective and highly specific immune response against the antigen.

The restriction of T cells to recognise antigens only when they are associated with either class I or class II MHC molecules is tied up with the fact that T cells do not bind to *intact* or 'native' antigen molecules—unlike B cells, which do. T cells recognise *fragments* of antigen, and so antigens must first be *processed* by other leukocytes and then *presented* to the T cell before activation can take place.

3.3.4 Antigen processing and antigen presentation

B cells and phagocytic white cells, including macrophages and other members of the monocyte lineage—especially those known as **dendritic cells**—engulf antigenic macromolecules and cells. While the antigen is inside the cell it is broken down into fragments, which reappear on the cell membrane. This is known as **antigen processing**. The alterations in structure between the native antigen and the processed antigen are essential for T cell recognition, but the precise details of these changes have not yet been determined for any antigen. The processed antigen fragments associate in the cell membrane with either class I or class II MHC molecules, and in this form the antigen can be bound by the receptor of a T cell from the appropriate clone. The various types of white cell that can present processed antigen to T cells in this way are known collectively as **antigen-presenting cells** or APCs.

Any cell that expresses sufficient levels of the appropriate MHC molecules *may* be able to present correctly processed antigen to T cells, but it is not certain whether all immune cells are equally effective at both processing and presentation. A division of labour may occur in which the phagocytic immune cells carry out the main processing operation and then expel the antigen fragments. These may be picked up by B cells, become associated with surface-bound class II molecules and then be presented to the matching clone of T cells. This model has the merit of bringing helper T cells into close contact with B cells that require 'helper' signals before clonal expansion and antibody production can begin.

3.3.5 Cytokines and lymphokines

By now you will have understood that the immune system (both innate and adaptive) consists of a vast network of cells, which interact with each other by making transient contacts between receptors on the surface of one cell and ligands on the surface of, or secreted by, other cells. We will now briefly review a structurally and functionally diverse group of *secreted* molecules, which transmit signals between cells engaged in an immune response. These molecules are all single polypeptides with a very short 'range' (i.e. they do not circulate in the body fluids as antibodies do) and a very short half-life (a few minutes in some cases). In effect they are *hormones* with specialised functions in regulating the immune response, and they are known collectively as **cytokines** (from the Greek *kineo*, to move, and *cytos*, a cell).

☐   Which cytokines have already been mentioned in this Book?

■   The interferons (which enhance NK activity) and chemotactic factors (which attract white cells) are mentioned in Chapter 2. Earlier in Chapter 3 we mentioned helper factors secreted by helper T cells, which are essential for the activation of most clones of B cells.

Those cytokines that are synthesised and secreted by small lymphocytes are known as **lymphokines**, and most of these are made by T cells. Between them, the lymphokines contribute to the activation or suppression of every cell in the immune system. It follows that for each lymphokine there must be a receptor with a complementary shape on the surface of the responding cell. We will describe some types of lymphokine in a moment, but first we must go back a step and ask what signals a T cell requires *before* it will secrete its lymphokines.

All three main subsets of T cells require binding of their matching antigen in association with certain MHC molecules. In addition, all three require activating signals from other cells *after* the antigen-plus-MHC has been bound by the T cell receptor. Cytotoxic T cells and suppressor T cells get their additional activating signals from lymphokines secreted by *helper* T cells; helper T cells get their additional activating signal from a cytokine secreted by *macrophages*. Macrophages in contact with any antigen secrete a protein known as **interleukin-1** or **Il-1**, which has a general growth-promoting action on helper T cells (and also on B cells). Note that the term 'interleukin' denotes a chemical signal transmitted between leukocytes. Helper T cells cannot synthesise and secrete the numerous different lymphokines that activate many other cells in the immune response without first binding to Il-1. Il-1 is also a potent inducer of fever by acting directly on the mechanisms in the hypothalamus that regulate body temperature. This has the indirect effect of enhancing T cell activity: T cells express more surface receptors and secrete more lymphokines when human body temperature rises, up to about 39 °C.

All helper T cells that have been activated by antigen-plus-MHC *and* Il-1, secrete at least 20 different lymphokines—sometimes referred to as 'helper factors'—with a wide range of functions and target cells (Figure 3.11 and Table 3.2). It is possible that some of these lymphokines are *antigen specific*, that is, they act only on cells in contact with the *same* antigen that activated the originating T cell. But most are *antigen non-specific* and can act on immune cells in contact with *any* antigen. Another group of lymphokines stimulate immature leukocytes to differentiate into competent immune cells, and other lymphokines are toxic to their target cells.

As you study Table 3.2, a word of caution needs to be expressed about the details shown. The names given to lymphokines are changing all the time, as laboratories around the world discover that two apparently different lymphokines are in fact the same molecule or, conversely, that properties attributed to one lymphokine are shared by another. Inevitably, different names exist for the same molecule, and although attempts at standardisation are proceeding, the nomenclature is not yet uniform. Several of the most important lymphokines synthesised by helper T cells have recently been redesignated as interleukins and given Il-numbers, which are shown in Table 3.2 along with the earlier descriptive names. But even this designation can lead to confusion since the first molecule to be called an interleukin (Il-1) is secreted by *macrophages* and is therefore *not* a lymphokine!

By means of the different lymphokines that they secrete, helper T cells are able to 'switch on' the adaptive immune response, increase its rate and intensity, and boost the effectiveness of the innate response. Also, by activating the *suppressor* T cells when the response has achieved its effect, helper T cells initiate the reduction of the immune response, thereby limiting the damage caused to 'bystander' tissues. Suppressor T cells inhibit the action of other immune cells by synthesising and secreting their own lymphokines, which are sometimes referred to as 'suppressor factors'. Helper and suppressor T cells are two of the most important sources of regulation of the immune response; these and other regulatory mechanisms are discussed further in Chapter 9.

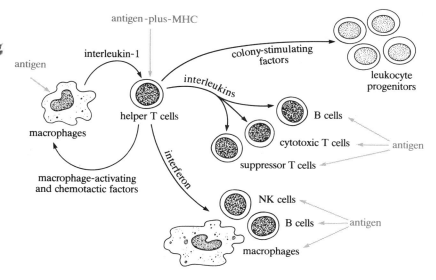

FIGURE 3.11 Activation of helper T cells requires contact with antigen-plus-MHC *and* a chemical factor called interleukin-1 (Il-1), which is secreted by macrophages in contact with antigen. Once activated by these signals, helper T cells secrete numerous chemical factors (collectively known as *lymphokines*), which activate most other immune cells in contact with antigen. Antigen alone is a weak or insufficient activator of the immune response.

TABLE 3.2   Some major lymphokines secreted by helper T cells

Lymphokine	Target cell(s)	Action
antigen-specific helper factors (T_HF)	T cells and B cells of the correct clone	promote proliferation and differentiation into active immune cells
interleukin-2 (Il-2)	all T cells and B cells	promotes proliferation
B cell growth factors, stimulation factors and differentiation factors (Il-4, Il-5 and Il-6)	all B cells	promote proliferation and differentiation into antibody-secreting cells
migration inhibition factor (MIF)	macrophages	prevents macrophages from leaving infection site
macrophage activation factor (MAF)	macrophages	activates
chemotactic factor (CF)	phagocytes	attracts
interferons (particularly γ-interferon, IFN γ)	NK cells	promote killing of virus-infected cells
	macrophages	activate
	B cells	promote proliferation and differentiation
colony stimulating factors (including Il-3)	progenitors of monocytes, granulocytes and red cells	promote growth and differentiation
lymphotoxins (including tumour necrosis factor, TNF β)	non-leukocyte target cells (especially tumour cells)	cytotoxic

35

3.4 T cell and B cell traffic through the body

We conclude this Chapter with some diagrams of the immune system that will enable you to trace the routes that T cells and B cells take in their journeys around the body and discern how they are brought into physical contact with each other, with the cells involved in the innate response, and with antigens. Figure 3.12 shows the **primary lymphoid organs**—the bone marrow and the thymus—in which B cells and T cells (respectively) differentiate from multipotent stem cells, and the *secondary* or **peripheral lymphoid system**, in which they spend the great majority of their active lives. The peripheral lymphoid system includes encapsulated organs, such as the spleen, tonsils and lymph nodes, and unencapsulated diffuse lymphoid tissue in the gut, urinogenital tract and lungs, in which white cells of many different types are densely packed together. The lymphatic vessels and their finely-branched ends, the lymphatic capillaries, form a network throughout the body that is at least as extensive as the vascular system. This network connects the body tissues to the lymph nodes and other lymphoid organs (Figure 3.13).

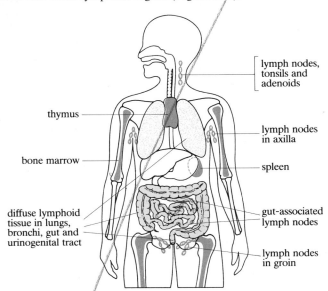

FIGURE 3.12 Distribution of lymphoid organs and tissues in the human body. The thymus and bone marrow (in red) constitute the *primary lymphoid organs*, so called because immature small lymphocytes differentiate into their mature, immunologically competent form in these organs. All other lymphoid organs and tissues, plus the lymphatic vessels, which form a network between them (Figure 3.13), constitute the secondary or *peripheral lymphoid system*, in which the mature small lymphocytes circulate.

The lymphatic vessels contain a fluid called **lymph**, which drains into the lymphoid organs from nearby tissues. Lymph originates as *plasma* leaking from the finest blood capillaries. Water and small molecules are transported across the walls of the lymphatic vessels and capillaries and returned to the bloodstream, so the lymph becomes more protein-rich as it moves through the system. Antigens entering the body at any point are rapidly swept towards a lymphoid organ. Each of the lymphoid organs filters fluid from a particular part of the body: the spleen filters the bloodstream, the lymph nodes filter the lymph draining from the intercellular spaces, and the diffuse lymphoid tissues filter lymph from the gut, lungs and urinogenital organs. There is no pump equivalent to the heart in the lymphatic circulation: lymph is agitated, rather than pumped around the system, by the smooth muscular walls of the vessels and the flexing and relaxing of striated muscles as the person moves around. All lymph eventually arrives at two large lymph *ducts* which empty into major veins in the neck, restoring the fluid and proteins to the venous circulation.

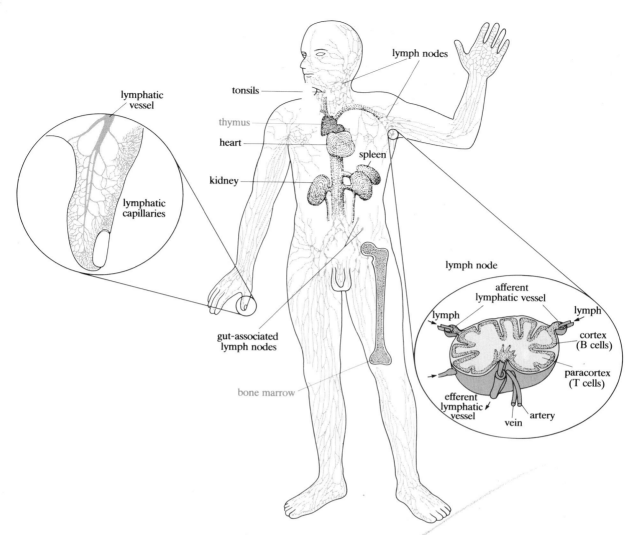

FIGURE 3.13 The human lymphoid system, showing the primary lymphoid organs in pink. The inset of the thumb illustrates the extent of the lymphatic capillary network. The inset of a cross-section through a lymph node identifies areas that are populated mainly by B cells or T cells. Lymphatic vessels carrying lymph *into* a lymph node are called *afferent* vessels, and those carrying lymph *out* of a lymph node are called *efferent* vessels.

The lymphoid system is the main territory in which the adaptive immune response takes place and, as you might expect, some lymphocytes spend most of their lives circulating around it. The lymphatic circulation contains predominantly the memory T and B cells and the naïve T cells (naïve B cells are very short-lived and remain in the lymphoid organs). Figure 3.14 shows the route of circulation of lymphocytes through the lymphoid system, into the bloodstream via the thoracic duct, and out of the venous capillaries to rejoin the lymphatic circulation as it passes through the tissues and lymphoid organs. Plate 3.2 shows lymphocytes migrating through the walls of the finest venous capillaries (known as high endothelial venules) in a lymph node. As you study Figure 3.14 you should bear in mind that lymphocytes spend only a few *minutes* in the bloodstream during each circuit, compared with several *hours* in the lymphoid system. Lymphocytes can also be found migrating through the body tissues. Macrophages and other phagocytic antigen-presenting cells, such as the dendritic cells, spend most of their lives migrating through the tissues until they encounter antigen, which is then phagocytosed and transported to the nearest lymph node.

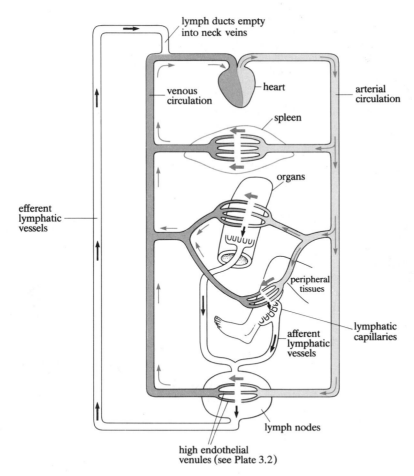

FIGURE 3.14 Circulation of lymphocytes through the mammalian lymphoid and vascular (red) systems. Afferent lymphatic vessels carry lymphocytes, lymph and antigens from the organs and tissues to the lymph nodes; efferent lymphatic vessels return lymphocytes and lymph to the vascular circulation in the neck. Lymphocytes re-enter the lymphoid system from the bloodstream either in the tissues or by migrating through the walls of specialised venous capillaries (the *high endothelial venules*, or HEV) as they pass through the lymph nodes (Plate 3.2).

Lymphocytes circulate through the body until they encounter the antigen for which they have appropriate receptors. If antigen is bound in the tissues, then the main consequence is an acute inflammatory response in which T cells participate directly, and to which antibodies contribute as described earlier. Antigen binding in the lymphatic or vascular circulation stimulates lymphocytes to migrate to the nearest lymphoid organ and stay there, and when antigen reaches a lymph node there is a rapid and profound decline in the number of cells leaving the node.

☐   What is the value of activated lymphocytes becoming stationary in a local lymphoid organ?

■   If they continued to circulate they would be moving away from the site of infection; and by settling in a local lymphoid organ they are brought into close proximity with other lymphocytes committed to recognise the same antigen, and with the antigen-presenting cells that are essential for T cell function.

The detailed internal structure of the peripheral lymphoid organs is beyond the scope of this Book, but they share a characteristic anatomical feature in that T cells and B cells are concentrated in different parts of the organ, with macrophages and other antigen-presenting cells clustered around these T cell or B cell areas (see detail of lymph node in Figure 3.13). Activated B cells also migrate back into the bone marrow and differentiate into plasma cells there; perhaps 80 per cent of the antibodies generated during a secondary response arise from plasma cells in bone marrow.

The anatomy of the lymphoid and vascular systems thus enables lymphocytes to patrol the tissues and the vessels forming the highways of the body. It also holds them in antigen 'traps' in the lymph nodes and other lymphoid organs, and brings them into close proximity with other immune cells, which is essential for the cell-to-cell communication that recruits, directs and regulates a coordinated response.

Summary of Chapter 3

1 Small lymphocytes exist in clones; the cells of each clone have antigen receptors in their surface membranes that bind to a particular epitope. A clone is 'selected' when a lymphocyte of that clone binds to its complementary antigen; this event initiates clonal expansion and the formation of effector and memory cells.

2 B cells mature mainly in the bone marrow. The B cell receptor for antigen is surface immunoglobulin (sIg), which binds to native (intact) antigen.

3 After contact with antigen, most B cells differentiate into plasma cells, which synthesise and secrete antibodies that bind to the stimulating antigen. Each B cell can only produce antibodies with receptors for a *single* epitope (or at most a few structural analogues of that epitope).

4 Some polymeric antigens activate B cells independently of T cells, but most B cells require activating lymphokines from helper T cells before clonal expansion occurs.

5 The secondary antibody response starts more quickly, reaches a greater concentration, and persists much longer than the primary antibody response.

6 Antibodies bound to antigens activate, focus and enhance the mechanisms of innate immunity, including phagocytosis, NK activity and the acute inflammatory response. They may also block active sites on antigen molecules.

7 T cells in three main subsets mature in the thymus. Helper and suppressor T cells regulate the intensity and duration of the adaptive response, and influence the innate response, through the lymphokines that they secrete; cytotoxic T cells kill infected body cells. Some helper T cells are also involved in prolonged inflammatory reactions.

8 All T cells are restricted to recognising antigen only when it is in association with MHC molecules, which are found on the surface of virtually all body cells. The T cell receptor for antigen binds to the MHC molecules and antigen simultaneously.

9 T cells do not bind to native antigen, but only to fragments of antigen that have been processed by antigen-presenting cells and then transported to the cell membrane. Cells capable of presenting antigen to T cells include macrophages, B cells and phagocytic cells in the skin, lymphoid organs and tissues.

10 Helper T cells in contact with antigen must also bind to an activating protein secreted by macrophages, called interleukin-1 (Il-1), before they can undergo clonal expansion. Activated helper T cells secrete over 20 types of lymphokine, which contribute to the activation of all the other cells in the immune system.

11 The lymphoid organs and tissues are the principal sites for the adaptive immune response. They trap activated lymphocytes and antigens and bring them into contact with each other and with antigen-presenting cells.

Now attempt SAQs 8–13, which relate to this Chapter.

CHAPTER 4
THE MOLECULES OF ADAPTIVE IMMUNITY

In this Chapter we discuss the biochemical structures of three of the most important molecules or, more correctly, molecular assemblies in the immune system. We aim to show you that these molecules are pivotal in adaptive immunity and that their structures underlie their functions. We also aim to demonstrate their 'family' relationship by revealing structural, functional and genetic similarities between them, which shed light on the evolution of the immune response.

4.1   Molecules involved in antigen recognition

The three assemblies of molecules that we will be discussing in this Chapter are all involved in the recognition of antigen by B cells and by T cells. They are *antibodies*, or *immunoglobulin* molecules; the *major histocompatibility complex* (MHC) molecules; and the *T cell antigen receptor*. You were introduced to all of them in the previous Chapter, so you should have a clear idea of the parts they play in the adaptive immune response. However, the biochemical *structures* of these molecules hold the key to understanding how they achieve their precise *functions*. Moreover, the studies of structural biochemistry (especially of antibodies) led to a break-through in genetics when it was discovered that these complex molecules are encoded by DNA from widely separated parts of the genetic material by rearranging a relatively small number of genes or their mRNA transcripts. Note that there are hundreds of types of molecule involved in adaptive immunity (for example, the many different lymphokines listed in Table 3.2), but we will focus here on the three vital molecular assemblies that have the ability to combine selectively with antigens.

4.1.1   A little history

The history of research into the molecules that bind to antigens is a long and illustrious one, and we have not the space to tell much of it here. Decades of patient and unrewarded struggle precede most of the news-making discoveries in any branch of science. Immunologists have known of the existence of antibodies, MHC molecules and antigen receptors on immune cells since at least the 1930s, and informed speculation about their existence was around long before that. But we still don't have all the answers, although much progress has been made. As always in science, the major breakthroughs had to wait until technological innovations enabled new methods of investigation to be tried. In particular, the techniques of protein-sequence analysis, genetic engineering and gene sequencing, cell and gene cloning, and the development of pure preparations of antibodies with identical binding sites for a single antigen (called *monoclonal antibodies*—see Chapter 7) have been fundamental to recent progress in immunology.

Antibodies, also known as *immunoglobulins*, are the best characterised of the three molecular assemblies that we shall discuss. (Note that 'antibody' describes what the molecule *does*, i.e. it acts against foreign bodies, and 'immunoglobulin' describes what the molecule *is*, i.e. a globular protein involved in immunity.) Antibodies are the antigen receptor molecules found in the surface membrane of B cells and, unlike the MHC molecules and the T cell antigen receptor, they are also secreted in large quantities by plasma cells. This has enabled concentrated preparations of antibodies to be collected from serum, and also from the urine of people with a certain B cell tumour, who excrete huge quantities of antibodies or antibody fragments. The first experiments to isolate and purify antibodies were performed in the 1950s and 60s, and resulted in the Nobel Prize for Physiology or Medicine in 1972, shared by the British immunologist Rodney Porter and his American colleague Gerald Edelman. In 1988, a Nobel prize was awarded to the Japanese biochemist Susumu Tonegawa for the breakthrough that he and his team achieved in the 1970s on understanding the structure of the genes that code for immunoglobulins. Although we know a great deal about the structure of antibody molecules, we are still learning about their molecular genetics and the regulation of gene expression.

By contrast, our knowledge about the molecules of the *major histocompatibility complex* began in the 1930s, with experiments showing that grafts between different strains of inbred mice were rejected because the graft recipient recognised certain molecules on the cells of the graft as antigenic. These antigens were MHC molecules. Progress in elucidating their structures, genes and physiological functions in life (as opposed to the contrived situation of tissue transplants) was not made until the 1970s, and this work is still not complete. However, in October 1987 a major advance was achieved when a group led by Pamela Bjorkman and Don Wiley in the USA succeeded in crystallising one of the human MHC molecules and identifying the part of the structure that associates with the antigen before presenting it to the T cell receptor.

Most recently of all, it took until the mid 1980s before we had even a partial description of the *T cell antigen receptor*, a structure that had eluded description until then despite 20 years of research and speculation. Several groups from around the world succeeded in unravelling part of this complex structure in 1984, and all of them published simultaneously in the 8 March issue of the journal *Nature* amid tremendous excitement. A group led by Ellis Reinherz in the USA used sequence analysis of fragments of the receptor, which were identified by antibodies that they had raised against the receptor; Tak W. Mak in Canada and Mark Davis in the USA cloned, respectively, the human and the mouse genes that code for part of the receptor. Since these advances, more components of the receptor have been identified and more genes have been cloned, but we are still some way from a complete picture.

We now have a good basic understanding of all three of the molecular assemblies that recognise antigen. This enables us to compare their structures and the genes that encode them, and to see that they probably have a common evolutionary origin.

4.2 The antibody molecule

A general plan of the antibody molecule was given in the previous Chapter (Figure 3.5). The arrangement of the polypeptides from which it is made is shown in Figure 4.1. The two identical **heavy chains** are polypeptides of M_r 50 000–77 000, linked together by disulphide bonds and each linked to one of an identical pair of **light chains** of M_r 25 000. The molecule has two, essentially different, functions: part of the structure of the two **Fab** regions is complementary to, and hence binds with, a particular epitope; parts of the structure of the single **Fc** region are complementary to ligands or receptors in certain tissues, on immune-cell membranes (e.g. phagocytes), or in the first component of the complement cascade. Thus, antibodies have *recognition* functions and *effector* functions localised in different parts of the molecule.

The representation of the antibody molecule in Figure 4.1 has become the conventional shorthand for antibody structure, and we will use it throughout this

Book, but you should recognise the gross structural simplification involved. Figure 4.2 shows a more realistic space-filling model of a particular *class* of antibody molecule, known as *immunoglobulin G* (antibody classes will be discussed later in the Chapter). Notice the **hinge region**, which contributes to the great flexibility of the molecule by allowing the distance between the two *antigen binding sites* to vary and considerable rotation of the Fab regions relative to one another to occur.

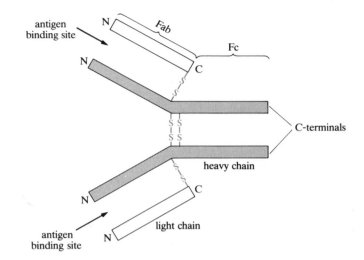

FIGURE 4.1 The structure of an antibody molecule. Note the disulphide bonds linking each light chain to a heavy chain, and joining the two heavy chains together.

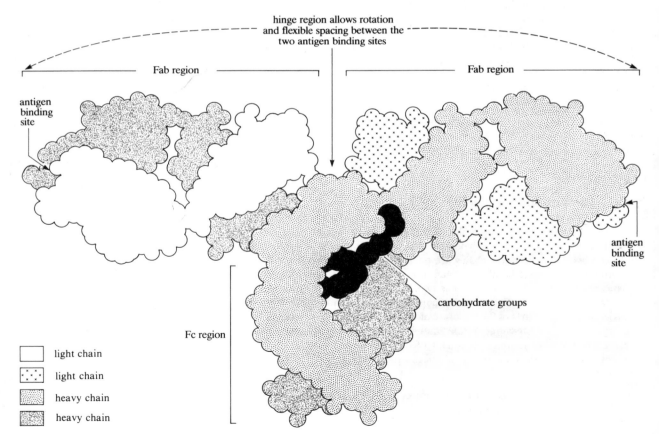

FIGURE 4.2 Schematic diagram of a space-filling model of an antibody molecule (immunoglobulin G = IgG). The heavy and light chains spiral round each other, making contact through opposing hydrophobic regions. The two heavy chains are held apart by the carbohydrate groups in the hinge region.

☐ What functional significance can you see for the flexibility of the antibody molecule?

■ Identical antigens (say) on the surface of a pathogen are unlikely to be a fixed distance apart, nor is their separation likely to be the same as some fixed distance between the two antigen binding sites on the same antibody molecule. Flexible spacing between, and rotation of, the antigen binding sites maximise the ability of the molecule to bind with *both* binding sites to antigens, and hence increase the *affinity* of the antibody for the antigen.

Molecular flexibility is especially important for cross-linking antigens on adjacent macromolecules or pathogens, because it enhances the phagocytosis of such aggregates (Figure 4.3). Soluble macromolecules may precipitate out of solution if large enough aggregates are held together by antibodies.

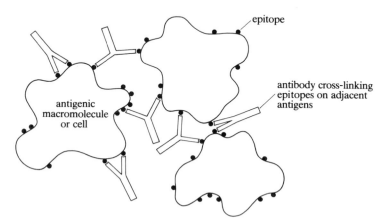

FIGURE 4.3 The flexible hinge region enables each antibody molecule to bind to epitopes that are various distances apart. This increases the ability of antibodies to *aggregate* antigen molecules or pathogenic cells into large clumps by linking adjacent antigens together (known as *cross-linking*). Aggregates of antigen are more easily eliminated by the mechanisms of innate immunity.

4.2.1 Constant and variable regions

Protein sequencing of the heavy and light chains of hundreds of antibody molecules that bind to different antigens, or nucleotide sequencing of their mRNA transcripts, has revealed that there is considerable *sequence variability* at the N-terminal end of the chains. Consequently, these regions of the light and heavy chains have been termed the **variable regions** (Figure 4.4). Conversely, the C-terminal ends of both light and heavy chains of different antibody molecules show considerable *sequence similarities*, regardless of which antigen they combine with. These parts of the molecule have been termed the **constant regions**.

☐ How does this *structural* division reflect the *functional* divisions of the molecule?

■ The variable regions correspond to the parts of the molecule involved in antigen recognition; each antibody molecule binds to an epitope with a particular conformation and thus requires a complimentary structure. The constant regions correspond to the parts of the molecule involved in effector functions common to most antibodies, such as binding to phagocytes or triggering the complement cascade by binding the first component.

The tertiary structure (higher-order folding pattern) of both the variable and the constant regions reveals a repeating pattern of *structural domains*. Light chains have two domains—one in the variable region and one in the constant region;

heavy chains have either four or five domains—one in the variable region and three or four in the constant region (Figure 4.4). Domains in the variable region of either type of chain are termed **variable domains** because their amino acid sequence varies between antibodies with different antigen specificities, even though their tertiary structures are very similar. Domains in the constant region of either chain are termed **constant domains** because they are similar in both primary *and* tertiary structure in different antibodies. However, as you will see later, there are small differences in the structure of the constant domains, which form the basis for dividing antibodies into five *classes*.

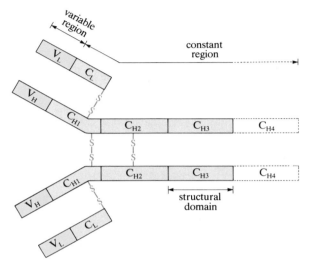

FIGURE 4.4 A schematic representation of an antibody molecule showing regions of highly variable or relatively constant amino acid sequences. The variable regions of both chains (V_L and V_H) each contain a single structural domain, as does the constant region of the light chain (C_L); the constant regions of the heavy chain (C_H) contain several linked domains (C_{H1} to C_{H4}). Some classes of antibody have three structural domains in the constant region of the heavy chain, and some have four.

All the domains (variable and constant) consist of two antiparallel *β-pleated sheets* stabilised by a single *intra*-chain disulphide bond running perpendicular to the plane of the sheets. Figure 4.5 shows the tertiary structure of the single variable domain (V_L) and the single constant domain (C_L) of a light chain. Notice that in the variable domain there are three *hypervariable loops*, which form the light chain's contribution to one of the antigen binding sites in the intact antibody molecule.

4.2.2   The antigen binding site

Each antigen binding site is formed from **hypervariable loops** in the variable domains of a pair of heavy and light chains. The hypervariable loops were discovered in the 1970s by protein-sequence analysis of a large number of variable domains from antibody molecules that bound to different antigens. The original analyses were carried out by the American immunologist Elvin A. Kabat and his colleague Tai Te Wu, a mathematical biophysicist. Their work revealed three hypervariable clusters, each of ten to 15 amino acid residues, in the heavy-chain variable domain, and three smaller clusters in the light-chain variable domain (Figure 4.6).

X-ray crystallography has since confirmed that the amino acids occupying these hypervariable positions create six loops (three in each chain). Their size, shape,

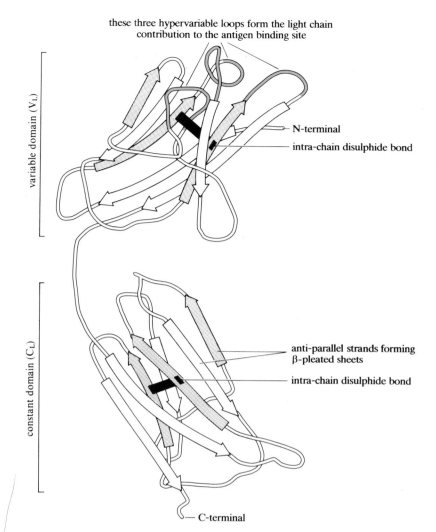

these three hypervariable loops form the light chain
contribution to the antigen binding site

variable domain (V_L)

N-terminal

intra-chain disulphide bond

constant domain (C_L)

anti-parallel strands forming
β-pleated sheets

intra-chain disulphide bond

C-terminal

FIGURE 4.5 Tertiary structure of the variable and constant regions of an antibody light chain, showing the two structural domains (V_L and C_L). The arrow-heads show the direction of folding of the polypeptide chain back and forth in antiparallel strands that form two β-pleated sheets in each domain (the three strands in one direction are shaded and the other three are white). Three loops in the chain at the tip of the variable domain (red) show *hypervariability* in their amino acid sequence when antibodies of different antigen specificities are compared. The variable domain of each heavy chain (not shown here) also has three hypervariable loops.

charge profile and distribution of hydrophobic groups is unique and precisely combines with the complementary surface of the antigen. This part of the antigen's surface is called the *epitope* (Figure 4.7).

The exact *shape* of the antigen binding site is (as you would expect) extremely variable, and depends on the precise *sequence* of amino acids in the hypervariable loops. Some binding sites are barrel-shaped clefts, but others are not deeply indented. The *size* of the binding site in the few antibodies that have been crystallised is up to 3.0 nm across and 2.0 nm deep. A binding site of this size could make contact with an epitope of about five to seven amino acid residues or perhaps three or four sugar residues. Epitopes are thus very small areas of much larger macromolecules: antigens found in nature have a relative molecular mass of at

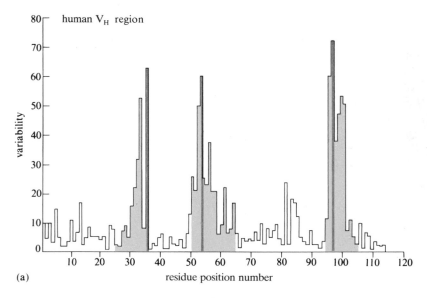

(a)

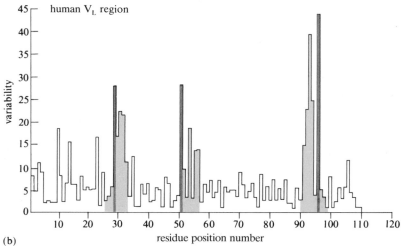

(b)

FIGURE 4.6 Hypervariable amino acid positions (red) in the primary structure of the variable region of (a) heavy chains and (b) light chains of human immunoglobulins. The data are the pooled results of hundreds of sequence analyses on antibodies with different antigen-binding specificities. Variability is calculated from the number of *different* amino acids found in a particular position, divided by the frequency of the most *common* residue found in that position. The residues in the shaded positions determine the complementarity of the binding site for a particular epitope.

least M_r 1 000, and most are much larger than this, regardless of whether they are part of an infectious organism, a surface component of a body cell, or 'free' in the body fluids. (We return to the nature of antigens and epitopes in Chapter 6.)

Molecules with a M_r below 1 000 are not usually able to elicit an immune response, even if they have epitopes in their structure, unless they are first attached to a larger 'carrier' molecule. Small molecules that contain epitopes are known as **haptens**. Haptens illustrate an important but often confused point of terminology: they are **antigenic**, i.e. they have epitopes in their structure that will combine with antibodies or T cell receptors with a complementary shape, but they are not **immunogenic**, i.e. they are not capable of provoking an immune response unless

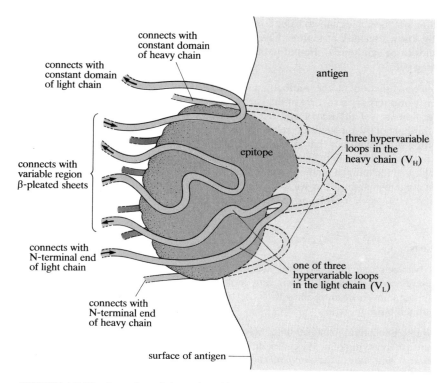

FIGURE 4.7 The formation of the antigen binding site by six loops of polypeptide (three each in the heavy- and light-chain variable domains) that have a hypervariable amino acid sequence when antibodies of different antigen specificity are compared. The amino acids in the hypervariable loops define the precise size, shape, charge and position of hydrophobic or reactive groups in the binding site, and hence determine the conformation of the epitope to which the antibody can bind.

they are attached to a larger molecule. The likely reason for this is that small molecules are completely broken down during antigen processing, so the epitopes are destroyed. If a hapten is linked covalently to a large molecule, enough epitopes survive processing to be presented to T cells and elicit a specific immune response.

Figure 4.8 shows three molecules of one such hapten, 2,4-dinitrophenol (2,4-DNP), attached to a large carrier molecule, bovine serum albumin (BSA). On their own, molecules of 2,4-DNP do not provoke an immune response when injected into laboratory animals (they are *not* immunogenic). But antibodies with binding sites for 2,4-DNP epitopes can be elicited by linking the hapten covalently to BSA and injecting the hapten–carrier conjugate into an appropriate recipient. Antibodies formed as a result will bind to 2,4-DNP molecules even when they are *not* linked to the carrier (the hapten alone is *antigenic*).

Affinity labelling studies using chemically-reactive haptens have provided important information about the structure of the antigen binding site, and have led to the identification of precisely which amino acids are involved in the recognition of a few, well characterised epitopes. Haptens normally form only *non-covalent* bonds with the amino acids in the binding site, but chemically-reactive haptens can be activated (for example by ultraviolet light) to form *covalent* bonds. If the polypeptide chains forming the variable domains of the light and heavy chains are then 'unravelled' by denaturation, the amino acid residue (or residues) bound to the hapten can be located and identified. In a few cases, particular residues at

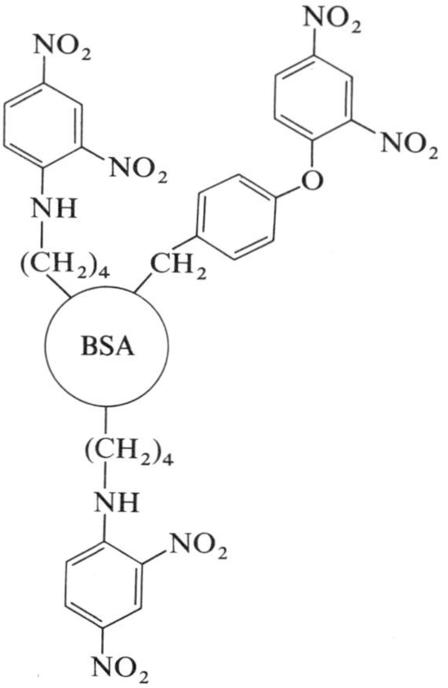

FIGURE 4.8 A typical hapten–carrier conjugate. Three haptens, each containing a 2.4-dinitrophenyl group (2,4-DNP), are linked to a bovine serum albumin (BSA) carrier molecule. Each of the 2,4-DNP groups contains an epitope to which complementary antibodies will bind. (Not drawn to scale: the BSA carrier is very much larger than the haptens.)

47

particular locations in the antigen binding site have been shown to be essential for antigen recognition. Haptens with fully known tertiary structures have enabled computer models of antigen binding sites to be synthesised. Bound haptens have also been co-crystallised with the binding site.

In summary, then, the antigen-*recognition* function of the antibody molecule resides in the precise amino acid sequence and tertiary structure of the part of the molecule at the tips of the N-terminal domains of the heavy and light chains. Extreme variability in the structure of this part of the molecule corresponds to the extremely diverse biochemical composition of the epitopes that the organism may be exposed to throughout life. Later, we turn to the ways in which the enormous diversity of antibody structure in the region of the antigen binding site is coded for by the *immunoglobulin genes*. But first we must discuss the ways in which the structure of the *Fc region* of the antibody molecule enables it to carry out its *effector* functions.

4.2.3 Antibody classes and their functions

The differences in antigen specificity between one antibody and another are located in the Fab regions of the immunoglobulin molecule. We will now look at differences in the Fc region, which can occur even in antibodies with the *same* antigen specificity (i.e. with identical antigen binding sites).

Five **classes** of antibody have been characterised on the basis of differences in the *constant* region of the *heavy* chains. There are five types of heavy chain, differing in the number of *constant* domains, the number and sites of the *disulphide bonds* that hold the four chains together, the number and location of *carbohydrate groups* attached to the heavy chains, and the relatively small variations in the amino acid *sequence* within the constant domains. The five types of heavy chain have been given the Greek letters γ (gamma), α (alpha), μ (mu), δ (delta) and ε (epsilon), which correspond to the Arabic letters G, A, M, D and E. Antibodies are divided into five classes on the basis of which of these chains they contain. Antibody classes are thus termed immunoglobulin G (IgG, pronounced *eye-gee-gee*), immuno-globulin A (IgA, *eye-gee-ay*), immunoglobulin M (IgM, *eye-gee-em*), and so on.

Within the IgG and IgA classes, further small differences in heavy-chain structure have enabled a number of *subclasses* to be distinguished. Although all mammals produce antibodies of all five classes, different subclasses have been found in different species, indicating that some subclasses have evolved *after* speciation has taken place. The classes also go further back in evolution than the mammals: IgG is found in birds, and antibodies that most closely resemble IgM have been found in the most primitive fish.

Table 4.1 summarises some of the major physico-chemical and functional charac-teristics of the five immunoglobulin classes of human antibody; these will not be repeated when we briefly discuss each class. Notice from Table 4.1 that in three of the classes (IgG, IgD and IgE) the antibodies always exist as *single* molecules, or **monomers**, but in the other two classes (IgA and IgM) the antibody molecules commonly *polymerise*. The **valency** of an antibody refers to the number of antigen binding sites in the most abundantly occurring form, be it monomeric or polymeric.

Immunoglubulin G

IgG forms by far the most abundant class of antibody in human serum. It is not produced in quantity until the *secondary* response, so its abundance reflects the extent to which we are continually defending ourselves against common patho-gens. The domain structure of IgG is shown in Figure 4.9, which also indicates the most important effector functions and the domains that are responsible for them. The monomers of other classes of immunoglobulin (not shown) are constructed according to the same basic plan, but with variations in the number of constant domains and disulphide bonds.

TABLE 4.1 Characteristics and functions of the human immunoglobulin classes

immunoglobulin class	IgG	IgA	IgM	IgD	IgE
heavy-chain type	γ	α	μ	δ	ε
number of constant domains in each heavy chain	3	3	4	3	4
relative molecular mass (M_r) of monomer	150 000	160 000	180 000	185 000	200 000
normally found as polymer?	no	dimer	pentamer	no	no
valency: number of antigen binding sites in normal form (i.e. monomer or polymer)	2	4	10	2	2
percentage of total immunoglobulin in serum	70–80	13–20	6–10	0–1	0.002
serum half-life (days)	23	5.8	5.1	2.8	2.3
ability to trigger complement cascade*	+ +	—	+ + +	—	—
can cross placenta from mother to foetus*	+	—	—	—	—
binds to Staphylococcal cell walls*	+	—	—	—	—
binds to macrophage Fc receptors*	+	—	(+)?	—	—
binds to neutrophil Fc receptors*	+	+	(+)?	—	—
binds to mast cell and basophil Fc receptors	—	—	—	—	+ + +
binds to platelets	+	—	—	—	—

* For IgG this refers only to some subclasses.

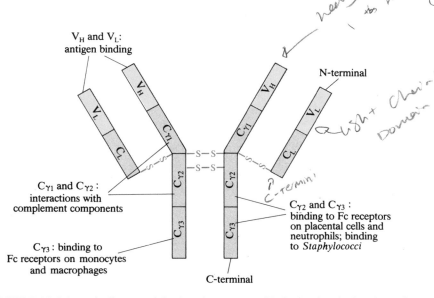

V_H and V_L: antigen binding

N-terminal

$C_{\gamma 1}$ and $C_{\gamma 2}$: interactions with complement components

$C_{\gamma 2}$ and $C_{\gamma 3}$: binding to Fc receptors on placental cells and neutrophils; binding to *Staphylococci*

$C_{\gamma 3}$: binding to Fc receptors on monocytes and macrophages

C-terminal

FIGURE 4.9 Schematic diagram of the domain structure of IgG, showing the functions of each domain. The C_γ domains are unique to IgG and, though very similar to each other, small structural differences confer specialised functions on this part of the molecule. Note that the four chains are held together by four *inter*chain disulphide bonds.

IgG diffuses through the walls of blood vessels more readily than the other classes and is thus the major class found in tissue fluids. It can also diffuse across the placenta and is found in colostrum and breast milk, so it has a vital role in the passive protection of new-born babies from infection (*passive* because the antibodies originate from the mother, not the baby). Its ability to bind to Fc receptors on phagocytic cells and to activate the complement cascade gives it a major role in the opsonisation of bacteria and the acceleration of local inflammatory reactions.

Immunoglobulin A

The main function of **IgA** is to protect the exposed surfaces of the body from pathogens, particularly bacteria and fungi. IgA is found predominately not in serum but in the mucus and watery secretions bathing the mucous membranes lining the body surfaces that are in contact with the outside world; thus, saliva, tears, sweat, nasal secretions and mucus in the lungs, gut and urino-genital tract are rich in IgA. Plasma cells found close to these membranes synthesise **dimers** of IgA (Figure 4.10 and Plate 4.1), which consist of two IgA monomers connected by a polypeptide of about 15 000 M_r called the **J chain**. The dimers are secreted by the plasma cells and are then taken up by epithelial cells in the mucous membrane. The epithelial cells add another component to the dimer, known as the **secretory piece**, before secreting it into the extracellular fluids bathing the membrane.

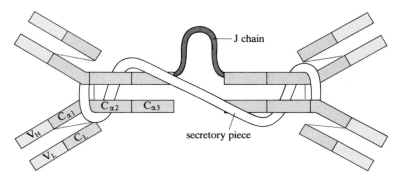

FIGURE 4.10 Schematic diagram of two IgA monomers joined in the dimer conformation by a *J chain* attached by disulphide bonds (not shown) to the $C_{\alpha3}$ domains of two IgA heavy chains. The secretory piece is added by epithelial cells *after* the dimer has been secreted by the plasma cell; it winds around the dimer and is attached by disulphide bonds (not shown) to the $C_{\alpha2}$ domains. The secretory piece is essential for transport of the dimer across mucous membranes. Disulphide bonds joining the light and heavy chains of IgA are shown as red lines.

☐   IgA dimers have a valency of four. Would you expect the four antigen binding sites of the IgA dimer to combine with different epitopes?

■   No. The two monomers are joined by the J chain *inside* the plasma cell. Each plasma cell can synthesise antibodies with only one antigen specificity, so all four binding sites must be identical. This enables the dimer to cross-link (aggregate) molecules of the same antigen more efficiently, although in practice all four binding sites are not always able to 'reach' epitopes.

Immunoglobulin M

IgM is found almost exclusively in serum and it is the first and most abundant class of antibody to be secreted into the circulation during the *primary* response to an antigen. Monomers of IgM are the predominant class of surface immunoglobulin (sIg) that is carried in the membrane of 'naive' B cells as their antigen receptor. IgM in serum is normally found as a **pentamer**, i.e. a polymer of five monomers connected through their Fc regions by disulphide bonds and a molecule of J chain

(Figure 4.11). The valency of the IgM pentamer is therefore ten. Electron microscope photographs of the pentamer (Plate 4.2) show that it adopts a star shape when unbound, but that flexibility in the junctions between the five monomers allows it to become crab shaped so that many of the binding sites can make contact with the antigen. In practice, it is rare for all ten binding sites to be filled because the probability of ten identical epitopes occurring 'within reach' of the binding sites is low.

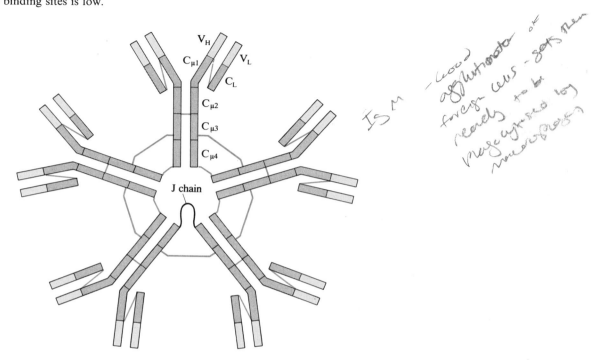

FIGURE 4.11 Schematic diagram of an IgM pentamer formed from five monomers of IgM, two of which are joined at the $C_{\mu 4}$ domains by a molecule of *J chain*. However, the pentamer is stabilised mainly by disulphide bonds (shown as red lines) between adjacent $C_{\mu 4}$ domains and by others joining the $C_{\mu 3}$ domains. (IgM and IgE are the only classes of immunoglobulin to have four constant domains in the heavy chain.)

☐ Given this structure, what particular function would you predict for IgM?

■ The high valency of the IgM pentamer enables it to form many cross-links between adjacent molecules of the same antigen. (Another way of saying this is that IgM pentamers *agglutinate* antigens.) As you know from Chapter 3, *aggregates* of antigen are more readily disposed of by phagocytes.

Immunoglobulin D

The function of **IgD** remains obscure. It is predominately found bound to the surface of B cells at a certain stage of their development, in association with surface-bound IgM monomers, so it may be involved in antigen recognition. Another hypothesis is that it is involved in maintaining B cell *tolerance* to molecules on the surface of the body's own cells. It is particularly susceptible to proteolytic enzymes, which may explain its very short half-life in serum.

Immunoglobulin E

Only traces of **IgE** are found in serum because antibodies of this class are almost exclusively found bound by the Fc region to the surface membrane of basophils and mast cells. IgE is thus localised mainly in the skin, lungs, and mucous membranes of the body. IgE antibodies are particularly likely to be synthesised in response to antigens on non-pathogenic plant or animal cells (or their debris) that are airborn and hence commonly breathed into the respiratory tract. IgE antibodies are also formed in response to certain chemicals in contact with the skin, and to certain foodstuffs.

☐ Can you predict what might occur when one of these antigens binds to the appropriate IgE antibodies attached to basophils or mast cells?

■ The cell degranulates, causing a local acute inflammatory reaction.

IgE antibodies are the major antibody class involved in allergic inflammatory (or *hypersensitivity*) reactions to non-infectious antigens (*allergens*), such as pollens, house-dust mites, food proteins and certain chemicals in contact with the skin. The reaction is an unfortunate side-effect of the evolutionary role of IgE as a precipitator of inflammatory reactions around parasites that have invaded the body. Allergies and other sorts of hypersensitivity reactions are discussed in the final Chapter of this Book.

4.2.4 Antibodies are also antigens!

Before we leave the structure of the antibody molecule and all its variations, a further point needs to be made. Each antibody monomer is a complex protein with a M_r of up to 200 000, and with a high degree of variability in its primary and higher-order structure, at least in parts of the molecule. It should not surprise you, therefore, to learn that *epitopes* exist in the structure of antibody molecules. Some of these epitopes are not immunogenic in the species in which the antibody was synthesised, but they *are* immunogenic if the antibodies are introduced into another species. Thus, for example, mouse antibodies are recognised as *antigens* if they are injected into a rabbit, and the recipient will mount an immune response, which includes the synthesis of rabbit antibodies with binding sites for epitopes on the mouse antibodies.

You may have a little more difficulty in accepting that some of the epitopes on an antibody molecule are immunogenic *in the animal that synthesised the antibody*. These epitopes are referred to as **idiotopes** (from the Greek *idios*, meaning 'own'). We will discuss the significance of idiotopes fully in Chapter 9, but for the moment you should note that within a given individual, *anti-idiotypic* antibodies that have binding sites for idiotopes exist. Put another way, we make antibodies against our own antibodies! These interlocking networks of antibodies are an important element in the control mechanisms that regulate the nature and intensity of the immune response.

4.3   The immunoglobulin genes

We turn now to the genes that encode immunoglobulins, and review the important contribution that an understanding of antibody genetics has made to the revolution in thinking about genes and their products. The pioneering work of Susumu Tonegawa on **immunoglobulin genes** in the 1970s dismantled two basic genetic precepts: that 'one gene codes for one polypeptide' and that 'the genome of somatic cells is constant'.

Tonegawa was aware that plasma cells produce antibodies of a *single* antigen specificity, yet between them they were capable of producing tens of millions of specificities. According to the basic precepts of genetics in the early 1970s, each B cell must contain all the genes necessary for manufacturing all these different antibodies, but only one set of immunoglobulin genes is expressed in each cell. There is an obvious flaw in this reasoning. The number of antigen specificities in the antibody repertoire of a human is estimated to be about 10^8, and each antibody molecule has a M_r of at least 150 000. The mass of DNA needed to code for 10^8 structurally different proteins of this size would be about 2.5×10^{-9} g, but the mass of DNA per human cell is only about 5×10^{-12} g. Thus, if a B cell were to contain the genetic codes for all antibodies it would require around 500 times the actual DNA content of the cell.

Tonegawa and his colleagues made a profound breakthrough in genetics by demonstrating three things. First, that a relatively small number of immunoglobulin genes are *recombined* in individual B cells during development, so each mature B cell expresses a unique combination of immunoglobulin genes, which encode an antibody molecule with a unique structure and hence a particular antigen specificity. Second, that many of the immunoglobulin genes that are *not* expressed in a particular mature B cell have been excised from the DNA (i.e. the DNA content of somatic cells is not constant). Third, that the genes that remain are found on *different* chromosomes in widely separated clusters, so their products (mRNA transcripts) have to be spliced together to make the heavy and light chains of the antibody molecule. All of these findings were highly controversial when they were first published in the 1970s, but Tonegawa was awarded the Nobel Prize for Physiology or Medicine in 1988 for his contribution to modern-day understanding of genetic recombination and RNA processing.

4.3.1. The generation of antibody diversity

Since Tonegawa's original work, many laboratories have contributed information to the picture that we now have of the genetic reorganisation that goes on as B cells differentiate from so-called *germ-line cells*, which contain all the genetic information that was present in the DNA of the zygote (the fertilised ovum from which the embryo develops). However, we still have some way to go in discovering the mechanisms that govern these genetic events.

In the germ-line cells, there are three sets of **germ-line genes** involved in immunoglobulin coding: one set codes for the heavy chains, and the other two code for two types of light chain designated by the Greek letters **kappa** (κ) and **lambda** (λ),which differ significantly in the amino acid sequence of their constant domains. The three sets of germ-line genes (*heavy-chain*, and κ and λ *light-chain* genes) occur on three different chromosomes in human cells, and also in mouse and rat cells (the only other species characterised so far). Each chromosome exists in a pair, one inherited from the maternal parent and one from the paternal parent; thus, there are two alternative versions of each of these three gene sets. In any given B cell only one chromosome of each *heavy-chain* pair expresses its immunoglobulin gene set. Moreover each B cell can synthesise *either* kappa light chains *or* lambda light chains, but never both—transcription of *one* chromosome from either set inhibits transcription of the other *three* chromosomes that have *light-chain* genes in that cell. The process by which heavy- and light-chain expression is reduced to one gene set of each type per cell is known as **allelic exclusion**.

☐   What is the consequence of allelic exclusion? (Hint: think about the structure of the antibody molecule.)

■   If, for example, both chromosomes in the pair containing the *heavy-chain* genes expressed these genes, then two *different* heavy chains would be synthesised by the same cell—one encoded by the paternal *heavy-chain* genes and one by the maternal genes. This could result in three different combinations of heavy chain in the finished antibody molecule (i.e. maternal/maternal; paternal/paternal; and maternal/paternal). The same would be true for the light chains. Allelic exclusion also ensures that hybrid antibody molecules with one κ and one λ light chain never occur in life. Expression of only one *heavy-* and one *light-chain* gene set ensures that all the antibody molecules produced by a B cell at a given stage of its development are identical, and thus have binding sites for the same antigen and display the same effector functions.

Although each B cell synthesises antibodies with either kappa or lambda light chains, but never both, in the B cell population as a whole, some cells express the *kappa* genes and others express the *lambda* genes, so both types of antibody molecule can be found in the circulation. Humans synthesise about twice as much kappa immunoglobulin as lambda, but different ratios exist in other mammals (e.g. the kappa:lambda ratio is 25:1 in mice but 1:25 in horses).

Figure 4.12 shows the location and approximate number of genes within each of the three germ-line sets in human cells. The **V, J**, and **D genes** code for the *variable* regions of the antibody molecule (J stands for 'joining' and D for 'diversity'), and the **C genes** code for the *constant* regions. Before describing the rearrangement of these genes during B cell development, we must unravel a contentious issue about terminology, which rests on the definition of a *gene*. If you accept the convention that one polypeptide chain is coded for by one gene, then each of the gene sets shown in Figure 4.12 should properly be considered as a *single gene* because each codes for a complete light or heavy chain polypeptide. The various alternative coding sequences within each set (V, J, D or C) should, according to this definition, be termed *gene segments*, since they are all parts of a single gene coding for one polypeptide. Unfortunately, immunologists have not been consistent in their use of terminology, sometimes referring to these alternative coding sequences as gene segments and sometimes simply as genes, often in the same sentence! In this book, we intend to take the simplest course and refer to each alternative V, D, J or C coding sequence as a *gene*, but you must be clear that by doing this we are moving beyond the old rule of 'one gene, one polypeptide'.

So, returning to Figure 4.12, notice that each of the three germ-line sets contains from two to at least 300 alternative V genes, together with a small number of alternative J genes, and that the heavy-chain set also has alternative D genes. Any

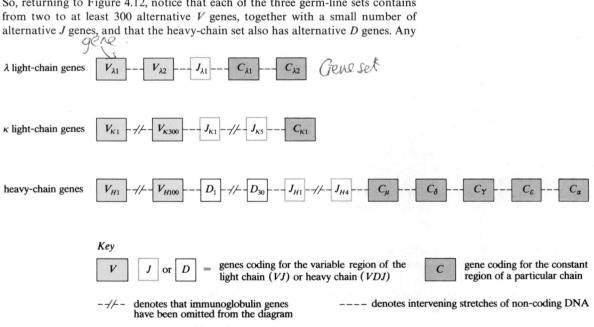

Key

| V | J or D | = genes coding for the variable region of the | C | gene coding for the constant |
| light chain (VJ) or heavy chain (VDJ) | | region of a particular chain |

--⁄⁄-- denotes that immunoglobulin genes have been omitted from the diagram

---- denotes intervening stretches of non-coding DNA

FIGURE 4.12 The three immunoglobulin gene sets in human germ-line cells, before somatic recombination. The number of alternative genes in the V_κ and V_H regions of the genome is not known exactly, so the numbers given should be taken as approximate. Note that these three gene sets are on three *different* chromosomes in the human genome and in the mouse genome.

of these genes can contribute to the variable regions of antibody molecules. Each set has from one to five alternative C genes coding for different constant regions. All the constant-region and variable-region genes are *continuous*, that is, each gene is a single sequence of coding DNA known as an *exon*. (Most genes are discontinuous, i.e. they are made up of several exons separated by non-coding sequences known as introns, which fall *within* the gene; it is interesting that the immunoglobulin genes each consist of a single exon without introns.) However, many of the genes are widely separated from each other in the DNA strand by non-coding sequences of nucleotides, which may be transcribed into mRNA but which are never translated into polypeptide.

As a germ-line cell differentiates into a mature but 'naive' B cell (i.e. one that is reactive to but has not yet encountered its matching antigen), **somatic recombination** of the germ-line genes takes place. In each cell, one of the V genes from each of the three germ-line sets is 'selected' by an unknown but probably random process, together with one of the adjacent J genes (and in heavy chains, also with one of the D genes). These selected genes are brought together in the genome when the *intervening DNA is excised*. It is not known whether the excised DNA and the genes that it contains are deleted altogether or transferred to other locations in the genome of the B cell. The basis of diversity in the antigen-recognition structure of an antibody molecule rests initially on this recombination event, since different genes are recombined in different B cells. Somatic recombination is sometimes referred to as *gene splicing*, for obvious reasons, but this term is easily confused with the artificial splicing of genes in genetic engineering; the word 'somatic' indicates the significant point that the genetic recombination takes place naturally in somatic (body) cells, not during gamete formation. Given the number of alternative V, J and D genes to choose from, you can see that a great many variations in the combination selected are possible.

☐ Using the numbers given in Figure 4.12, calculate the number of different combinations of V and J genes that are possible in the *kappa light-chain* germ-line set.

■ There are at least 300 different V_κ genes, any one of which could recombine with one of the five alternative J_κ genes. So there are $300 \times 5 = 1\,500$ possible combinations. In this way, a relatively small number of germ-line genes can produce at least $1\,500$ κ light chains, each with a structurally unique variable region, and hence a particular antigen specificity.

The recombination process in the heavy chain produces even more variation since there are at least 100 V_H genes, 30 D genes and four J_H genes to choose from ($100 \times 30 \times 4 = 12\,000$). The recombination events of the heavy and light chains are independent of each other, so any heavy chain can occur with any light chain. The antigen binding site of an antibody molecule is constructed from parts of both the heavy and the light chain, so the total number of different antibodies with κ light chains is $12\,000 \times 1\,500 = 18$ million! Somatic recombination is the first major source of variation in antibody structure and hence in antigen specificity, but there are other mechanisms that increase the variation still further, as you will see in a moment. First, however, we must follow through the sequence of transcription and translation of these recombined genes into a completed polypeptide chain.

The second line of Figure 4.13 shows the somatic recombination of the germ-line genes coding for a hypothetical κ light chain. When these recombined genes are transcribed into mRNA, further 'trimming' of the code occurs by a process known as *RNA splicing*. This is exactly analogous to the DNA splicing that occurs during somatic recombination. First, a *primary* mRNA transcript is made; this contains the code from the selected V gene, together with the transcript of all the remaining J genes, the C_κ gene and the non-coding sequences that separate them. The transcript is then cut and spliced to make a *mature* mRNA transcript, in which the 'excess' J genes and the non-coding sequences between the genes are excised. Thus, the mature mRNA only contains the code transcribed from a single V, J and C_κ gene, joined together in a linear sequence. The mature mRNA transcript is then translated into the κ light-chain polypeptide.

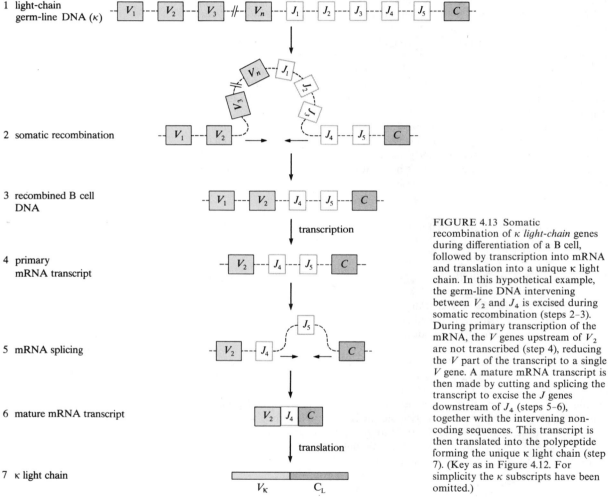

FIGURE 4.13 Somatic recombination of κ *light-chain* genes during differentiation of a B cell, followed by transcription into mRNA and translation into a unique κ light chain. In this hypothetical example, the germ-line DNA intervening between V_2 and J_4 is excised during somatic recombination (steps 2–3). During primary transcription of the mRNA, the V genes upstream of V_2 are not transcribed (step 4), reducing the V part of the transcript to a single V gene. A mature mRNA transcript is then made by cutting and splicing the transcript to excise the J genes downstream of J_4 (steps 5–6), together with the intervening non-coding sequences. This transcript is then translated into the polypeptide forming the unique κ light chain (step 7). (Key as in Figure 4.12. For simplicity the κ subscripts have been omitted.)

The process by which heavy chains are synthesised (Figure 4.14) is very similar to that described above. Somatic recombination of the germ-line genes results in a B cell with selected V, D and J *heavy-chain* genes brought close together by the elimination of most (but not all) of the intervening genes. Initially at least, there is no elimination of any of the five different *heavy-chain C* genes, each coding for the constant regions of one of the heavy-chain *classes*. Thus, each B cell is initially capable of producing antibodies of any of the five classes. However, all these antibodies have binding sites for the *same* antigen because, once selected, a *VDJ* combination is not altered by further recombination. As you will see in a moment, individual B cells at different stages of their lives do indeed produce antibodies of

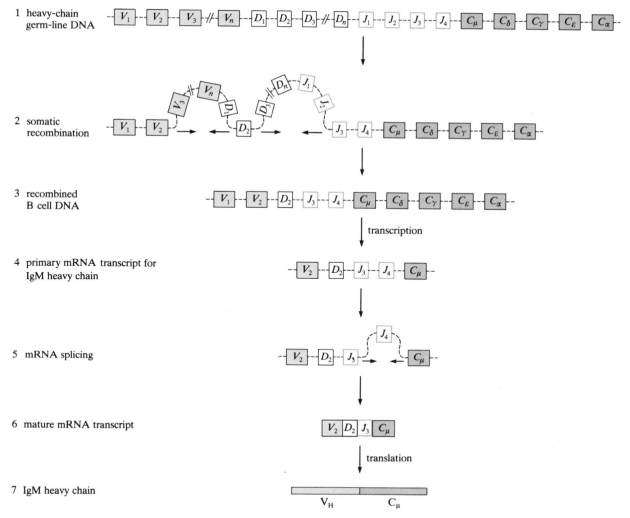

FIGURE 4.14 The formation of an IgM heavy chain with a unique variable domain. The sequence shows the somatic recombination of *heavy-chain* germ-line genes during differentiation of a B cell (steps 2–3), followed by transcription of *VDJ* genes and C_μ into a primary mRNA transcript (step 4), mRNA splicing to remove excess *J* genes and non-coding sequences (steps 5–6), and translation into an IgM heavy chain (step 7). (Key as in Figure 4.12. For simplicity, the *H* subscripts have been omitted.)

different classes but with the same antigen binding sites. In the example shown in Figure 4.14, the germ-line DNA intervening between V_2 and D_2 is excised, together with the DNA intervening between D_2 and J_3, to give the recombined B cell DNA. The primary mRNA transcript contains only the selected *VDJ* cluster, together with the transcript of the 'excess' downstream *J* genes, and the transcript of the first of the *C* genes, C_μ. The mature mRNA transcript is made by excising the excess *J* genes and the non-coding sequences, and this is then translated (in this example) into an IgM heavy-chain polypeptide.

Although the first source of variation in the structure of the antibody molecule is brought about by somatic recombination of alternative *V*, *D* and *J* genes, further diversity in the amino acid sequence of the variable domains results from **variable recombinations**, i.e. slight variations in the exact location of the 'cutting points' as first the germ-line DNA and later the mRNA transcripts are cut and spliced. Both these sources of variation occur *before* contact with antigen.

Yet more variation arises *after* contact with antigen. Single base changes occur in the DNA of activated B cells, mainly during the process of memory-cell formation.

This process is called **somatic mutation**. The *V*, *D* and *J* genes are particularly susceptible to mutations, which generate small but significant variations in the antigen-binding site. Together, the three major sources of variation (somatic recombination, variable recombination and somatic mutation) account for the enormous range of antigen specificities—at least 10^8 different antigen binding sites—that has been estimated to exist among the antibodies produced by a single individual.

Another consequence of somatic mutation is that some of the binding sites produced by the mutated DNA have a better *affinity* for the antigen, and some have a worse affinity. This is because the mutations occur randomly in the DNA coding for the variable region, sometimes improving the 'fit' between the antigen binding site and the epitope and sometimes reducing it. Somatic mutations occur mainly during memory-B cell formation, so the memory B cells from a single clone end up with receptors (i.e. surface immunoglobulin) for the *same* antigen, but with a *range* of antigen affinities.

☐   What effect will this have on the antigen affinity of the antibodies *secreted* during the secondary response, and why?

■   The affinity will be improved. This is because memory cells with the *higher-affinity* antibody in their surface membranes are *more likely* to bind the antigen at second exposure than are cells with the lower-affinity sIg. Thus, cells producing the higher-affinity antibody will be 'selected' for activation during the secondary response. This process is known as **affinity maturation**.

Changes in the *class* composition of the antibodies produced during an immune response also take place.

4.3.2   Immunoglobulin class switching

If you look back at the example given in Figure 4.14, you will notice that the first *C* gene downstream of the *VDJ* genes remaining in the B cell DNA is C_μ, the gene coding for the constant domains of heavy chains of the IgM class. Because transcription always takes place in one direction (from 5' to 3'), the primary mRNA transcript made from this DNA code contains the transcribed version of C_μ, and hence the resulting antibodies will be IgM. You should recall that antibodies of the IgM class act as the surface-bound receptor for antigen on naive B cells, and that IgM is the predominant class of antibody secreted by circulating B cells in contact with their matching antigen for the first time. Naive B cells (i.e. mature but not yet activated by antigen) *also* have surface-bound molecules of IgD. The cell can synthesise *both* IgM and IgD by transcribing both C_μ and C_δ, and then trimming the transcripts to remove the code for IgM heavy chains from some and the code for IgD heavy chains from others.

As the primary immune response proceeds, some B cells undergo further DNA recombination of the *C* genes. A number of routes for this recombination have been proposed, all producing the same result (Figure 4.15). Path (a) in Figure 4.15 shows one route in which C_μ and C_δ are excised from the DNA; path (b) shows an alternative route in which the mRNA transcripts of these genes are spliced out during production of a mature mRNA transcript. A third hypothesis (not shown) suggests that an additional C_γ gene is 'borrowed' from another part of the genome and is then spliced into the B cell DNA *upstream* of C_μ.

☐   What effect will the three alternative recombination routes described above have on the *class* of antibody synthesised by these B cells?

■   Because the C_γ gene is brought to lie immediately downstream of the genes coding for the variable region of the heavy chain, this gene will be transcribed into the mRNA and the cell will switch from synthesising IgM antibodies to synthesising IgG antibodies.

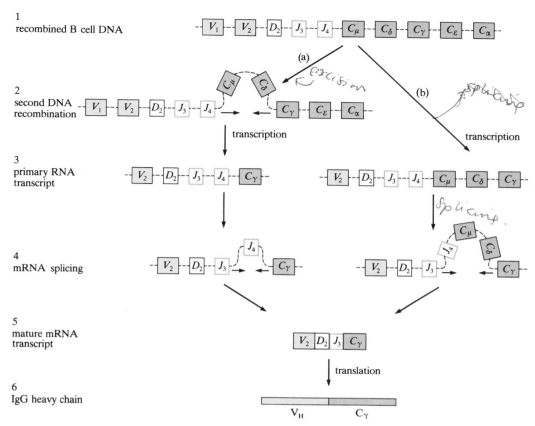

FIGURE 4.15 Heavy-chain class switching from IgM to IgG. The switching sequence shown in path (a) is *irreversible* because the genes for C_μ and C_δ are removed from the B cell DNA by recombination (step 2) before transcription to primary mRNA (step 3) and further mRNA splicing (step 4). The switching sequence in path (b) is *reversible* because all five C genes remain in the B cell DNA. Only the first three C genes are transcribed (step 3) and switching is achieved by excising the transcripts of C_μ and C_δ from the primary mRNA transcript (step 4). The result is the same for both paths: the mature mRNA transcript contains the codes for a unique *VDJ* combination together with C_γ. (Key as in Figure 4.12.)

Antibodies found in the serum during a *secondary* immune response are mainly of the IgG class, unlike those of the *primary* antibody response which are mainly IgM. This process is known as **class switching** and it occurs during the maturation of the adaptive immune response. Switches to produce the heavy chains of IgA and IgE probably occur in similar ways to those described above for the switch from IgM to IgG.

4.4 The major histocompatibility complex

The preceding discussion of immunoglobulin structure and genetics forms an excellent basis for understanding the way in which structure is related to function in the MHC molecules. As you will see, there are certain family resemblances which suggest that the present-day immunoglobulin genes and *MHC* genes may be descendants of a common evolutionary ancestor.

The existence of the MHC molecules (although not their nature) has been known since the 1930s, when their presence on red cell membranes was first demonstrated. Later experiments in the 1940s—catalysed by the need to develop successful skin grafts for burn victims of the Second World War—showed that organs or skin grafts transplanted between individuals from different strains of mouse were *rejected* because the recipient mounted an immune response against certain antigens on the cells of the graft. The molecules that the recipient responded to as antigens were originally termed *transplantation antigens*, but it is now recognised that they are the protein products of genes in the **major histocompatibility complex**. The **MHC molecules** are a group of membrane-bound glycoproteins concerned with cell-to-cell interactions in the immune response and, as you know from Chapter 3, they have been divided into two *classes*: class I and class II. Molecules in both classes consist of *two* polypeptide chains (i.e. a dimer) that are *dissimilar* and non-covalently linked, and one or both of these chains is anchored in the cell membrane. These molecules are therefore sometimes described as *transmembrane heterodimers*.

4.4.1 Class I MHC molecules

The generalised structure of the **class I MHC molecules** is shown in Figure 4.16b. The two chains are termed α and β. Only the α-*chain* of the two polypeptides in this dimer is coded for by genes in the *MHC* region of the genome. It consists of a polypeptide chain of M_r about 45 000, folded into three globular domains outside the cell membrane, which are attached to a short hydrophobic section traversing the membrane and a small hydrophilic section in the cytoplasm of the cell. It is often described as the class I heavy chain because the external globular domain nearest to the membrane (termed α_3) shows a striking similarity in primary and tertiary structure to the constant domains of immunoglobulin heavy chains. Like the Ig domains, the innermost domain of the class I α-chain is formed from two antiparallel β-pleated sheets (you can compare Figure 4.16a with Figure 4.5, which shows the tertiary structure of the constant domain of a light chain).

The α_1 and α_2 domains consist of short lengths of β-pleated sheet, topped by an α-helix. These domains include the epitopes that are recognised as foreign when tissue is transplanted between different individuals of the same species. However, it seems likely that the ability to recognise and kill cells in a tissue graft from a member of one's own species has arisen as a 'side effect' of the primary role of the cytotoxic T cell—namely, the killing of virus-infected cells that carry the 'self' form of the class I molecules. The α_1 and α_2 domains also include the region of the class I molecules that associates with the antigen in the cell membrane before it is 'presented' to a cytotoxic T cell. (As explained in Chapter 3, before the cytotoxic T cell can be activated, it must bind to an assembly of antigen plus class I MHC molecules.) Crystallographic studies have shown that a groove exists between the two outer domains of the α-chain (Figure 4.16a and c), which can accommodate an epitope of between eight and 20 amino acids. The class I molecules first bind to the antigen and then 'present' it to the cytotoxic T cell in a recognisable form.

The smaller chain of the class I molecules is known as the β-chain and consists of **β_2-microglobulin**, a small globular protein that (like α_3) is very similar to antibody constant domains in both tertiary structure and amino acid sequence. It is not inserted into the cell membrane, and is held to the α-chain by hydrophobic forces. (You may recall that hydrophobic forces also help to stabilise the positions of constant domains on adjacent heavy chains in the antibody molecule—see Figure 4.2.) The function of this polypeptide is not fully understood: it is certainly essential for stabilising the structure of the α-chain, but it may have other roles to do with antigen recognition or presentation that have not yet been discovered.

The human genome contains three major gene loci encoding class I molecules (as you will see in a moment when we discuss the *MHC* genes in more detail), thus each cell has up to three slightly different class I molecules on its surface. The antigen binding site in each of the class I MHC molecules must be capable of binding a huge variety of different antigens because the cell may become infected with any of a wide range of pathogens, each with unique antigens as part of its structure. In this respect, the binding of antigen by the MHC molecules is apparently far *less specific* than the binding of antigen by antibody molecules. However, further research is required before we can describe the exact details of how the MHC molecules bind to antigens, or delineate the extent of variation in the epitopes that can be bound by the *same* MHC molecules.

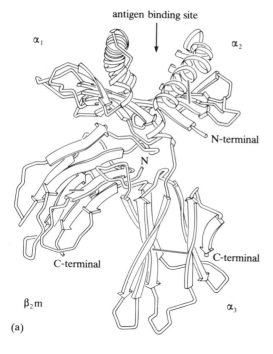

antigen binding site

α_1 α_2

N-terminal

N

C-terminal C-terminal

$\beta_2 m$ α_3

(a)

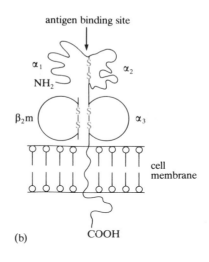

antigen binding site

α_1 α_2

NH_2

$\beta_2 m$ α_3

cell membrane

(b) COOH

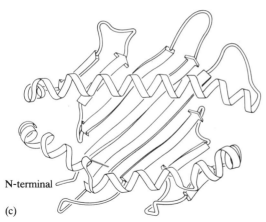

N-terminal

(c)

FIGURE 4.16 Structure of human class I MHC molecules. (a) Side view of a particular class I molecule (designated HLA-A2) as determined by crystallographic studies; other class I molecules differ in their primary structure in certain domains (principally α_1 and α_2) but are believed to have very similar tertiary structures to HLA-A2. Epitopes in the α_1 and α_2 domains are unique to each individual and are the principal targets for the immune response involved in transplant rejection. The antigen binding site is in a cleft between these two domains. (b) Stylised representation of the side view of human class I molecules, showing the orientation of the cell membrane. (c) Top-down view of the HLA-A2 molecule as determined by crystallographic studies, showing the cleft into which the processed antigen fits. The floor of the binding site is formed by short sequences of β-sheets, and the walls are formed by α-helices.

4.4.2 Class II MHC molecules

The generalised structure of the **class II MHC molecules** is shown in Figure 4.17. The class II molecules (like those of class I) consist of two dissimilar polypeptide chains, α and β; but in contrast with class I molecules, *both* chains are encoded by genes in the *MHC* region and *both* are inserted into the cell membrane. The α-chain has a M_r of 30 000–34 000 and the β-chain is smaller with a M_r of 26 000–29 000. Both chains have two globular domains outside the cell, attached to a short, hydrophobic transmembrane section with a hydrophilic section inside the cell. The domain that lies furthest from the cell membrane in each of these chains (α_1 and β_1) shows no sequence homology whatever with the immunoglobulin domains. But the domains closest to the cell membrane (α_2 and β_2) have significant structural similarities to the constant domains of immunoglobulin heavy chains.

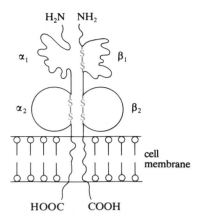

FIGURE 4.17 Stylised structure of the class II MHC molecules, showing two polypeptide chains (α-chain and β-chain) folded into four domains. The tertiary structure had not been determined by crystallographic studies at the time of writing (early 1989), but analysis of the amino acid sequence predicts a very similar structure to the class I molecules (Figure 4.16), with an antigen binding site in a cleft between the α_1 and β_1 domains. Epitopes in α_1 and β_1 are the targets for graft rejection reactions when tissue is transplanted to a non-identical recipient. The α_2 and β_2 domains resemble immunoglobulin heavy-chain constant domains.

☐ Which part (or parts) of the class II molecules would you expect to be involved in presenting antigen to *helper* T cells (as discussed in Chapter 3)?

■ The α_1 and β_1 domains are involved. They are suited to this partly because they lie outermost and are thus more accessible for antigen binding, but particularly because of their variable and unique structure, which enables them to combine with the variable and unique structure of different antigens.

Less is known at present about the antigen binding sites on class II molecules than those on class I molecules. However, analysis of the amino acid sequence and computer modelling predicts a very similar structure for a binding site in a cleft between the α_1 and β_1 domains. A further area of uncertainty concerns the role of class II molecules in restricting antigen binding by *suppressor* T cells. In mice we know that class II molecules present antigen to suppressor T cells, so it is possible that a similar process occurs in human suppressors. However, some human suppressor T cells have been shown to be 'guided' by class I MHC molecules rather than by class II molecules.

In the human *MHC*, three major gene loci encode the class II MHC molecules, so activated leukocytes may express up to three different class II molecules, in addition to the class I molecules, which occur on most cells in the body.

4.4.3 The *MHC* genes

The genes coding for the MHC molecules of both classes are on the *same* chromosome in human cells, but on a *different* chromosome from each of the three immunoglobulin gene sets and from the single gene coding for β_2-microglobulin. The primary structure of β_2-microglobulin is highly conserved; that is, molecules from different vertebrate species show a high degree of sequence homology.

☐ What does this suggest to you about the evolution of the gene that codes for this molecule?

■ It seems likely that it evolved in primitive vertebrates and has been passed on virtually unchanged as evolution has proceeded.

Similarities in the primary and higher-order structure of immunoglobulin domains and some domains in MHC molecules of both classes also suggest that all have descended from a common ancestral gene; however, they have diverged after duplication and been recombined to form complex functional gene sets as evolution has proceeded.

☐ What is the most obvious evidence of recombination of these genes?

■ They are on different chromosomes in present-day species.

Figure 4.18 shows the arrangement of major gene loci coding for the MHC molecules in humans and in mice. In humans these genes are known as the **HLA complex** (HLA stands for human leukocyte antigens, since the products of these genes are involved in recognition events between human leukocytes). In mice they are known as the **H-2 complex** (standing for *histocompatibility complex 2*, a title which reflects the involvement of MHC molecules in tissue graft rejection: *histos* is Greek for tissue).

The human *HLA complex* contains six major gene loci: three in the *D region*—*DP*, *DQ* and *DR*—which code for three different class II molecules, and *B*, *C* and *A*, which code for three different class I molecules. The mouse *H-2 complex* also has loci that code for either class I or class II molecules, but two additional class I

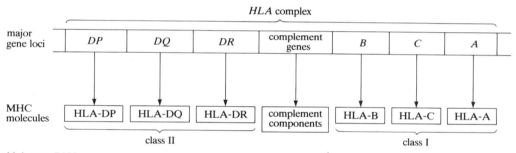

(a) human DNA

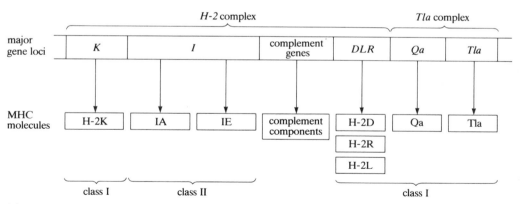

(b) mouse DNA

FIGURE 4.18 The *major histocompatibility complex (MHC)* genes and their products in (a) humans and (b) mice. Human *MHC* genes are termed the *HLA complex*, and mouse *MHC* genes are termed the *H-2 complex*. There are six major loci in the *HLA complex*, each coding for a different MHC molecule (three from class I and three from class II). Numerous alleles exist at each of the major loci, so the precise structure of each MHC molecule varies from individual to individual. In the mouse, some of the class I molecules are coded for by genes that lie downstream of the *H-2 complex* in the *Tla complex*; a human equivalent of these genes probably exists but has not yet been characterised.

molecules are encoded by genes that are *outside* the *MHC* region (in the adjacent *Tla* region). The products of the *I* region of the mouse *H-2 complex* (which contains two loci: *IA* and *IE*) are thought to have the same functions as the products of the *D* region of the human *HLA complex*—both are involved in determining how responsive a particular individual will be to a particular antigen (a subject to which we will return in Chapter 9).

Notice in Figure 4.18 that the genes in the *HLA complex* are organised in a different sequence from their equivalents in the *H-2 complex*. This is a further clue that ancestral genes have been recombined in different sequences in the two species to give these modern patterns. The *MHC* region of both species also encloses within it the genes encoding the components of complement, which seems to indicate that these genes have remained together through evolution. (Some texts refer to the complement genes as *MHC class III*, but the products of these genes have a totally different function from those of the class I and class II molecules, so this term may lead to confusion.)

A high degree of variability exists in the structure of individual *MHC* genes when different humans or mice are compared. Although the sequence of the major gene loci relative to one another never changes, the genes occur as numerous *alleles* (different forms). For example, more than 50 alleles of both the *H-2K* and the *H-2D* genes in the mouse *H-2 complex* have been identified, and a similar polymorphism exists in the human *HLA complex*. At each major gene locus only one of the possible alleles is inherited by a given individual. The number of different combinations of alleles is so far in excess of the number of individuals in the species that each individual has (theoretically) a unique combination of alleles at the major loci, and hence has a unique set of MHC molecules.

☐   How does the generation of diversity within the *MHC* genes differ from the way in which diversity is generated within the immunoglobulin gene sets?

■   Only *one* allele is inherited at each of the *MHC* loci, but *all* the alternative *immunoglobulin V* genes are present in the germ-line DNA. *MHC* diversity has already been achieved in the zygote, but immunoglobulin diversity arises during differentiation—or, put another way, *MHC* diversity is achieved at the level of the *population*, whereas immunoglobulin diversity arises in the *individual*.

Different individuals have different combinations of MHC molecules on their cells. Parts of the MHC molecules will be recognised as foreign antigens if tissues or organs are transplanted between individuals—even when the donor and recipient are members of the same family. Mismatches at certain of the major gene loci are more important than mismatches elsewhere in determining how 'foreign' the transplanted MHC molecules appear to the recipient's immune system, and hence how readily a graft will 'take' or be rejected. This explains the need for tissue typing. Only identical twins inherit identical *MHC* genes and hence have identical MHC molecules, and can thus freely accept tissue or organ grafts from each other.

Identical twins are **syngeneic**, i.e. genetically identical. Syngeneic laboratory rodents (particularly mice and rats) have been selectively bred over many years to give inbred strains in which all individuals are genetically identical *and* homozygous for all their genes. Some inbred strains differ from each other only in the allele present at a *single* identified locus; these strains are described as **congenic**. Inbred strains of rodent have proved to be tremendously important in unravelling the contribution of each locus in the *MHC* region to the ability of the animal to mount an immune response. For example, it has proved possible to evaluate the influence of particular alleles of genes in the *MHC* region on the effectiveness of cytotoxic T cell responses or helper T cell responses.

4.5 The T cell antigen receptor

The final piece in the antigen-recognition puzzle is the **T cell antigen receptor** which, as you know, must simultaneously be a receptor for the epitope of an antigen *and* for parts of the class I or class II MHC molecules, depending on which T cell subset is involved.

4.5.1 The structure of the receptor

The T cell antigen receptor has turned out to be another member of the immunoglobulin 'family' of molecules in that it also includes several domains with structural similarities to either constant or variable immunoglobulin domains (Figure 4.19). It consists of at least seven separate and different polypeptide chains inserted into the cell membrane and projecting into the cytoplasm. Only two of these chains make contact with the antigen and with the MHC molecules on the presenting cell; they are held together by a disulphide bond in a heterodimer known as **TcR** (which stands for *T cell receptor*; also referred to as *Ti* (*tee-eye*) in some texts). The commonest form of TcR on human T cells has an α-chain and a β-chain, each of M_r 40 000–45 000 and each with two domains. The outermost domain of each chain has a variable amino acid sequence when the receptors of T cells from different clones are compared. The precise sequence of amino acids in the TcR chains determines the antigen specificity of the T cell. Analysis of the primary structure of the outermost TcR domains predicts a folding pattern that is very similar to the folding of immunoglobulin *variable* domains. By contrast, the two domains closest to the cell membrane resemble the, by now familiar, heavy-chain constant domains of the immunoglobulins. A less common form of TcR has also been discovered in which the two polypeptides have been designated the γ-chain and the δ-chain; they have a similar structure to the more common α and β chains, and seem to be found most often on T cells in the skin. The significance of this is not known.

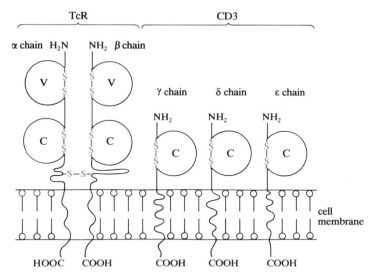

FIGURE 4.19 Schematic representation of five of the polypeptides forming the T cell receptor for antigen (in association with MHC molecules). The complex consists of two polypeptides known as TcR, which contain the antigen binding site in their variable domains (V), associated with at least five polypeptides (only three are shown here) known as CD3, which appear to be involved in signal transduction. The exact number and position of the CD3 chains in relation to TcR is not known (they may occur on *both* sides of TcR, as in Figure 4.21). Domains labelled C bear structural similarities to the constant domains of immunoglobulin heavy chains. Those labelled V resemble immunoglobulin variable domains.

Just as the antibody molecule contains *idiotopes* in its structure (i.e. epitopes that are immunogenic in the animal that synthesised the antibodies), so too the TcR chains contain idiotopes, which are recognised by anti-idiotope receptors on other immune cells or by anti-idiotope antibodies. Regulatory networks involving idiotope recognition are discussed in Chaper 9.

In addition to the TcR chains, the T cell receptor contains at least five polypeptide chains, which are non-covalently associated into a complex known as **CD3**. (Only three CD3 chains are shown in Figure 4.19; the precise number is not known, nor is the anatomical relationship between these chains and the TcR chains.) The CD3 complex appears to act as a *signal transducer*; it transmits the activation signal from the TcR chains, after they have bound to antigen-plus-MHC, to the cytoplasm of the cell. Signal transduction involves the calcium-dependent triggering of cyclic AMP production, which is a common form of transmembrane signalling in cells. The CD3 chains have an *invariate* structure from cell to cell, and they don't make contact with either the antigen or the MHC molecules on the 'presenting' cell; thus CD3 appears to perform an identical but essential function in all T cells, regardless of their subset or antigen specificity. It is yet another molecular complex that is structurally related to the immunoglobulins.

4.5.2 The *TcR* genes

The genes encoding the α- and β-chains of TcR were originally isolated by cloning genes that were expressed in T cells but not in B cells. This involved making DNA transcripts of mRNA messages found in active T cells and then seeing which of these *copy DNAs* (generally abbreviated to *cDNAs*) hybridised with B cell cDNAs and which did not. The cDNAs that failed to hydridise were unique to T cells. It turned out that the genes encoding the α- and β-chains are remarkably similar to the immunoglobulin genes. The region of the germ-line DNA that codes for all four types of TcR chain contains numerous alternative variable (V), diversity (D), joining (J) and constant (C) genes, which are recombined in different combinations as T cells differentiate from germ-line cells. Each mature T cell (like the mature B cells) has a unique combination of VDJ and C genes, thus coding for a unique antigen receptor. It has been calculated that there are at least 10^9 different VDJ combinations in the mouse genome, which is an order of magnitude *greater* than the number of T cells in the mouse's circulation. The diversity in human T cell antigen-receptor structures is even greater. However, the genes coding for the TcR chains are *not* prone to somatic mutation (unlike the immunoglobulin genes, which are), so there is no improvement in the affinity of T cell receptors for the complementary antigen as the immune response proceeds.

4.5.3 Interaction with antigen and MHC

Until the mid-1980s there were two competing models for the way in which the T cell receptor could achieve the simultaneous recognition of two entirely different molecules: antigen and the appropriate class of MHC molecule. One model proposed that the T cell receptor was in two distinct parts, one of which bound to the antigen and the other to the MHC molecule (the so-called *dual recognition* model); but evidence has been steadily growing that the other model, known as the **associative recognition** model, is correct. This model proposes that a *single* receptor exists, which binds to both the antigen *and* the appropriate MHC molecule. The TcR chains have the correct structural conformation to fulfil this task.

Figure 4.20 shows a schematic representation of the receptor of (a) the cytotoxic T cell and (b) the helper T cell, binding to antigen in association with the MHC molecules. The model is a theoretical one, based on predictions about the chemical structures of the polypeptides involved and their likely interactions. Notice that the surface marker molecules CD8 and CD4, which are found in the membrane of the cytotoxic and the helper T cell respectively (look back at Table 3.1), are involved in this binding event. CD8 interacts only with ligands in the class I MHC molecules,

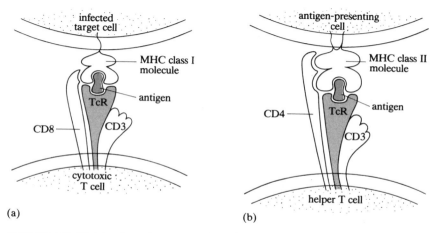

FIGURE 4.20 Highly schematic representation of theoretical receptor–ligand interactions at the cell surfaces of (a) a cytotoxic T cell and an infected body cell, and (b) a helper T cell and an antigen-presenting cell. The surface marker molcules, CD8 and CD4, for cytotoxic and helper T cells respectively, restrict the T cell to binding to MHC molecules of the correct class. CD3 is a complex of several polypeptides believed to be involved in signal transduction.

and CD4 only with ligands in the class II molecules. CD8 and CD4 therefore restrict T cells to bind only with the appropriate class of MHC molecule through the usual requirements for stearic complementarity between a receptor and its ligand. CD8 and CD4 also have domains in their structure that resemble the higher-order folding pattern (though not the primary structure) of the polypeptide chain in either constant or variable immunoglobulin domains (see Figure 4.21 in the following Section).

4.6 The immunoglobulin supergene family

We close this long Chapter by restating that the problem of accurate antigen recognition seems to have been solved by similar protein structures in at least three major molecular assemblies: the antibody molecule, the MHC molecules, and the T cell receptor molecules. Moreover, CD8, CD4 and CD3 are part of the same 'superfamily' of molecules, and as Figure 4.21 shows, the family does not end there.

At least two types of molecule involved in cell-to-cell *adhesion* have immuno-globulin-like domains (one of these, termed CD2, is shown in Figure 4.21), as do a number of molecules found preferentially on neurons and other cells in the brain (for example, the molecule known as *Thy-1*); cell-surface receptors for growth factors and receptors for the Fc region of antibodies are also part of the immunoglobulin 'family', and so is a polypeptide called *carcinoembryonic antigen* (CEA) which occurs only on embryonic cells and the cells of certain cancers. The function of some of these immunoglobulin-like molecules is unknown, but all of those with known functions are involved in receptor–ligand interactions at the cell surface that trigger a subsequent change in the activity of one or both cells in the interaction. Thus, the molecules of the immunoglobulin family have been tentatively attributed with adhesion or recognition functions.

The similarity in domain structure, and in some cases also in parts of the amino acid sequence, in these molecules strongly suggests that a 'supergene' existed at some point in evolution, and that it has since been copied, multiplied, mutated and recombined to give the many alleles of the *Ig, MHC, TcR* and other *Ig-family* genes that we see today. Although in many cases these genes occur in clusters on different chromosomes, they are unusual in that very few of them are discontinuous. The majority of the amino acid sequence for each *domain* in the immunoglobulins, the MHC molecules, the T cell antigen receptor and several other members of the

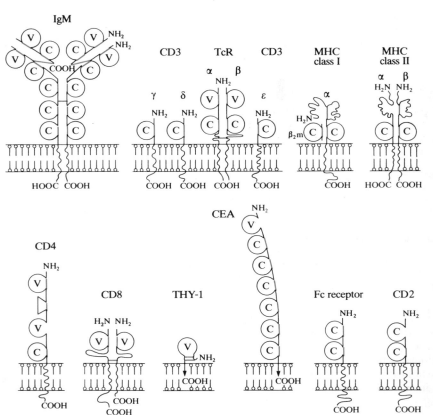

FIGURE 4.21 Products of the immunoglobulin supergene family. Regions resembling immunoglobulin domains have been drawn as circular loops, most of which are stabilised by an intrachain disulphide bond (shown in red). Those domains labelled V or C show similarities in their higher-order structure to immunoglobulin variable or constant domains respectively. See the text for a description of the functions of these molecules.

family, is encoded by a single *exon*, i.e. by a continuous sequence of coding DNA. This supports the notion that these 'blocks' of DNA have been shuffled around in the genome during evolution. Perhaps the definition of the relationship between genes and proteins should be recast as 'one gene codes for one domain'. The identification of the **immunoglobulin supergene family** has shed light on the general mechanisms by which genes evolve; other supergene families are already being identified.

This Chapter has described some of the most striking examples of cell-to-cell communication, and demonstrated that communication occurs as a result of non-covalent bonding between receptors on the surface of, or secreted by, cells and cell-bound or secreted ligands. The receptors and the ligands to which they bind are able to 'recognise' each other accurately amidst the background 'noise' of other cell-bound and free macromolecules solely because their higher-order structures include binding sites with complementary shapes. Some receptors pick up the antigen, others identify one cell type to another, still others distinguish the cell as 'self'. The necessity to generate a range of receptors, which between them can recognise and bind to millions of different antigens and specific cell-surface markers, has been met during evolution by the economical strategy of copying variations on (at most) a few ancestral genes.

Summary of Chapter 4

1   Three assemblies of molecules lie at the heart of adaptive immunity because they bind to antigen in a specific and selective way; they are the antibody molecule, the MHC molecules, and the T cell antigen receptor.

2   Specific antigen binding is achieved by all three of these recognition molecules in a similar way; part of their structure is highly variable in its amino acid sequence when a comparison is made between molecules synthesised by different cells

(antibodies and T cell receptors) or between molecules found on the cells of different individuals (MHC molecules). This polymorphism generates a range of receptors, each with binding sites for particular epitopes.

3   Other parts of these three molecular assemblies show a high degree of homology in higher-order and primary structure with the constant or variable domains of immunoglobulin heavy chains.

4   Many alternative immunoglobulin genes and T cell receptor genes exist in the germ-line DNA; diversity is achieved primarily by somatic and variable recombination of DNA, followed by mRNA splicing, as differentiation of B cells and T cells takes place. Both these families of genes exist as alternative V, D and J genes coding for the variable domains of the structure, and C genes coding for the constant domains.

5   The genes encoding the MHC molecules do not recombine in the individual; diversification is already present in the germ-line DNA as different alleles are inherited at each of several major gene loci.

6   The immunoglobulin, TcR and MHC molecules are each constructed from two or more dissimilar polypeptides assembled into a single molecular complex. These are held together by non-covalent bonds (particularly hydrophobic interactions) and, in the case of antibody and the TCR chains of the T cell receptor, also by inter-chain disulphide bonds.

7   The antigen binding site of the antibody molecule is formed by six hypervariable loops, three each in the polypeptide chains forming the variable domains of the light chain and of the heavy chain. The site can interact with an epitope of approximately three to seven amino acid or polysaccharide residues.

8   The antigen-affinity of the antibody molecules produced during the primary response is less than the affinity of secondary-response antibodies. Somatic mutations of the V, D and J genes during the formation of memory cells produce antibodies with a range of affinities for the same antigen; during the secondary response, antigen 'selects' those memory cells that have binding sites with the highest affinity to differentiate into antibody-secreting plasma cells.

9   Five classes of immunoglobulin exist (IgG, IgA, IgM, IgD, IgE), which differ in their heavy-chain constant domains and hence in their effector functions. The class of antibodies produced switches from mainly IgM during the primary response to mainly IgG during the secondary response. Class switching occurs through excising the heavy-chain genes for IgM and IgD from the memory-B cell DNA (irreversible class switching) or excising the transcripts of these genes from the memory-B cell mRNA (reversible class switching).

10   Epitopes exist in the variable regions of antibody molecules, and in the TcR chains, that are immunogenic within the individual that synthesised them. These immunogenic epitopes, or *idiotopes*, are involved in interactions with receptors on, or secreted by, other immune cells, and help to regulate the immune response.

11   MHC molecules include epitopes that are unique to the individual. This results in graft rejection when tissue is transplanted between individuals (unless they are identical twins or syngeneic rodents) but, more importantly, it restricts T cells to recognise antigens only when presented to them on the surface of the body's own cells.

12   MHC class I molecules are involved in the recognition of antigen by cytotoxic T cells; class II molecules are involved in the recognition of antigen by helper (and possibly some suppressor) T cells. Recognition requires binding of the appropriate MHC molecules to the processed antigen in an assembly, which then binds to the T cell antigen receptor and the appropriate T cell surface marker (CD4 or CD8). The T cell may be activated by a signal-transducing region of the receptor, known as CD3. (Note: other activating signals working through other receptors are also required, e.g. Il-1 or certain lymphokines; recall Chapter 3.)

Now attempt SAQs 14–18, which relate to this Chapter.

CHAPTER 5
COLLABORATION AND ESCAPE

In this Chapter we return to an overall view of the immune response, now that you have a more detailed knowledge of the individual mechanisms. We briefly review the ways in which innate and adaptive mechanisms rely on each other and collaborate in mounting a more effective immune response than either could achieve alone. But if this collaboration is so successful, why do we suffer from infectious and parasitic diseases at all? Part of the answer lies in the evolution of escape strategies by the organisms that are the targets for the immune response.

5.1   Collaboration between innate and adaptive immunity

The collaboration between innate and adaptive mechanisms is extensive and inevitable, given that they have evolved 'hand in hand'—in fact, the distinction between them has been emphasised largely for educational expediency! You should now be in a position to look back over the four preceding Chapters and review the points of contact between the two systems.

☐   In what ways does adaptive immunity *rely* on the functioning of innate immunity?

■   There are three main points of reliance. First, all subsets of T cells require processed antigens to be presented to them in association with the appropriate MHC molecules; antigen-presenting cells include macrophages and their close relatives in the monocyte cell lineage, such as dendritic cells, which are mediators of innate immunity. Second, *helper* T cells require an activating signal in the form of interleukin-1, which is secreted by macrophages in contact with antigen. Third, soluble chemotactic factors secreted by macrophages also attract T cells and B cells to a site of infection in the tissues.

☐   In what major ways does adaptive immunity *regulate* and *enhance* innate immunity?

■   There are many forms of regulation and enhancement: lymphokines secreted by helper T cells promote the proliferation, maturation and activation of all the cells involved in innate immunity, as well as attracting them to the site of an infection and immobilising them there; antibodies focus the mechanisms of innate immunity on to the targets to which they bind, promote phagocytosis by opsonisation and agglutination of antigens, and trigger the complement cascade and mast-cell degranulation and, hence, a local inflammatory reaction. Antibodies and interferons enhance or focus the killing power of innate cytotoxic cells, especially K and NK cells.

The interactions between the two systems form a positive feedback loop (until suppressor mechanisms come into play, of which more in a later Chapter). For example, activated macrophages secrete interleukin-1, which is essential for helper T cell activation; activated helper T cells secrete interferons, which are potent activators of macrophages. Interferons induce a significant increase in the expression of class II MHC molecules on the surface of macrophages, which in turn makes them more effective presenters of antigen to helper T cells. Figure 5.1 and Plate 5.1 demonstrate the effectiveness of collaboration between innate and adaptive immunity in the response to two very different infections.

However, innate and adaptive immune mechanisms collaborate not only by being mutually dependent in certain ways, but also by policing rather different *territories* and *targets*.

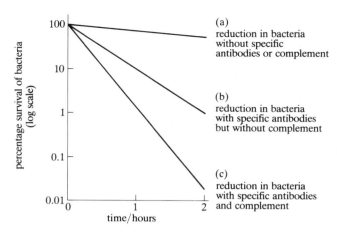

FIGURE 5.1 Collaboration between adaptive and innate immunity in eliminating bacteria from the serum of mice. In experiments (a) and (b), the mice were depleted of complement before bacteria were injected. In experiments (b) and (c), bacteria were incubated *in vitro* with antibodies that had binding sites for bacterial antigens and then injected into the mice. After two hours, there is more than a 1 000-fold decrease in the percentage survival of the antibody-coated bacteria in intact mice (c) compared with uncoated bacteria in complement-depleted mice (a).

5.1.1 Division of labour in the immune response

There are no hard-and-fast rules about which cells or mechanisms are effective against which targets or in which locations in the body, but some specialisation is evident. For example, the *tissues* of the body are mainly the province of tissue macrophages, complement, IgA and IgG (which, as you may recall, diffuses through blood vessel walls more readily than other classes of immunoglobulin). Pathogens in the *bloodstream* are subject to responses centred mainly on IgG and IgM, cytotoxic T cells and neutrophils, but remember that both IgG and IgM are potent activators of the complement cascade, so an inflammatory reaction will also contribute to immunity. Pathogens in the *lymphatic* circulation are controlled mainly by adaptive mechanisms rather than innate ones because lymphocytes are the main inhabitants of the lymphatic capillaries.

☐ Which cells or mechanisms would you expect to be the most important defences at the mucosal surfaces of the body, especially those lining the respiratory tract and the gut?

■ Specialised macrophages inhabit the lungs and migrate along the margins of the gut wall; IgA and lysozyme are found abundantly in mucus and inhibit the entry of pathogens (particularly bacteria) through the mucosa; IgE molecules become bound to the Fc receptors on the surface of mast cells below the mucosa, and cause degranulation if the antigen binding sites of the IgE are filled. Mast cell degranulation results in an acute inflammatory reaction, with all the attendant phagocytic cells and their toxic arsenal.

Just as there is a rough division of labour in terms of the relative importance of particular defence mechanisms at different *sites* in the body, so there are some variations in the effectiveness of those mechanisms against different *targets*. For example, circulating antibodies (mainly IgG and IgM) are most effective against *extra*cellular bacteria, whereas phagocytic and cytotoxic cells (T, NK and eosinophils) are most effective against *intra*cellular pathogens and protozoa. Eosinophils, mast cells and IgE offer the most effective defence against parasites that are too large to hide inside the body's own cells and too large for destruction by phagocytosis. Finally we should mention fungal infections, which are generally controlled very effectively by the mechanisms of innate immunity, particularly by the action of macrophages.

Thus, almost every part of the body is defended by a range of mechanisms directed against the many types of pathogen and parasite that may gain entry. (The healthy cornea is one exception because it has no blood or lymphatic supply; corneal grafts can therefore be transferred between non-identical individuals without rejection.) Defence mechanisms are also arranged in 'strata' in both space and time: if the first line of defence is penetrated, then others are brought into action, with an increasing concentration and specificity. But, despite the range and sophistication of the defence mechanisms that vertebrates have at their disposal, infectious and parasitic diseases persist, even in societies that have been able to afford adequate standards of public hygiene, housing, health education and nutrition. Why does the immune response fail to give complete protection?

5.2 Escape strategies

Pathogens and parasites have co-existed throughout evolution with the host organisms that they infect, and they are dependent on the survival of their target species to provide hospitality for future generations. The theory of *co-evolution* states that although natural selection favours adaptations in host organisms that protect them from pathogens and parasites, it also favours adaptations of the infectious organisms that will better enable them to survive in their hosts.

☐ In this competition, which side has the advantage and why?

■ Pathogens in particular, and multicellular parasites to a slightly smaller degree, have the enormous advantage of much shorter generation times than the hosts that they infect (for example, some bacteria have a generation time of only 12 minutes, compared with about 12 weeks for a mouse and at least 12 years for humans). Pathogens therefore evolve much faster than their hosts because advantageous mutations occur far more frequently and spread rapidly through the gene pool as a result of natural selection.

Pathogens and parasites have been able to evolve **escape strategies** that keep pace with or even outstrip the evolution of immune mechanisms in their hosts. But it is not in the long-term interests of the invading organism to make such a successful escape that the host is overwhelmed before another can be infected; if they did so, the most virulent pathogens would die out. So a state of *dynamic balance* exists (illustrated in Figure 5.2) between the host species and the species of infectious organism. The existence of this balance is demonstrated most forcefully when it is upset.

☐ Can you think of any examples to illustrate this?

■ AIDS is perhaps the most obvious contemporary example; normally innocuous infections become fatal when the immune system fails to function. You may also have thought of historical examples. The importing of a pathogen into a part of the world where it did not previously exist and where no defence against it had evolved has devastated entire communities (e.g. measles and other European infections killed hundreds of thousands of people in South America when the conquistadors invaded in the 15th and 16th centuries).

Another example is given by the enhanced virulence of a particular pathogen when it invades a host of a different species to its normal host. For example, rabies is regularly found in the fox population of mainland Europe without causing serious outbreaks of disease in the foxes (i.e. it is *endemic*); bubonic plague is endemic in rats; yellow fever is endemic in certain species of monkey; and brucellosis is endemic in cattle. But the infectious agents of all these diseases often produce fatal illness in human hosts, even though the original host displays a degree of resistance.

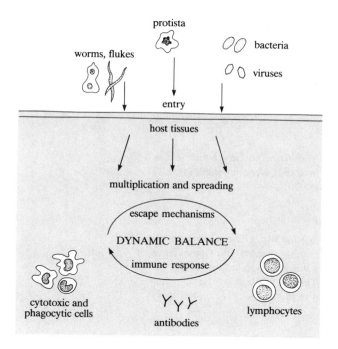

FIGURE 5.2 A dynamic balance exists between the evolution of more effective immune responses to pathogens and parasites, and the evolution of more effective escape strategies by these infectious organisms. Because of their short generation time, pathogens and parasites can adapt quickly to new defence mechanisms in their hosts, but if they become too successful their hosts will die out.

The escape strategies evolved by pathogens and parasites are as varied as the defences ranged against them, but some have proved especially successful. Bacteria, virus and parasite escape mechanisms have distinctive features, which we will discuss in turn.

5.2.1 Bacterial escape strategies

The list below is intended to illustrate the versatility of bacterial strategies. Notice that the causative agents of many important bacterial diseases in humans (such as tuberculosis, leprosy and pneumonia) are represented.

1 A few types of bacterial cell wall are resistant to enzymic degradation (e.g. by lysozyme), and *encapsulated* bacteria are particularly resistant to this defence.

2 Polypeptides in some bacterial capsules actively inhibit the attachment of phagocytes (e.g. the M-protein in *Streptococcus* species, or D-glutamic acids in the capsule of *Bacillus anthracis*, the causal agent of anthrax).

3 Some bacteria (e.g. *Bacillus anthracis*) secrete *toxins* that kill or repel phagocytes.

4 Other bacteria secrete *enzymes* that interfere with the host response in a number of ways. These enzymes may:

(a) inhibit the development of an inflammatory reaction at the site of infection (*Pseudomonas aeruginosa*, which causes diarrhoea, secretes an enzyme that inactivates C3a and C5a);

(b) spread the infection by breaking down the 'cement' between tissue cells (the enzyme *hyaluronidase* is secreted by some bacterial species);

(c) protect the bacterium by coating it with a layer of fibrin (*Staphylococcus aureus*, which causes abcesses in the skin, secretes a *coagulase* that does this);

(d) split IgA dimers into the less effective monomeric form (*Neisseria gonorrhoea*, *Streptococcus pneumoniae* and *Haemophilus influenzae* all secrete *proteases* that do this).

5 Some Gram-negative bacteria can inhibit the attachment of the membrane attack complex if the complement cascade is triggered.

6 Some bacteria resist destruction by phagocytes *after* they have been ingested:

(a) *Mycobacterium tuberculosis* is able to inhibit the fusion of macrophage lysosomes (which contain toxic molecules and oxidising agents) with the vacuole in which it was engulfed;

(b) *Mycobacterium leprae*, which causes leprosy, and *Legionella pneumophilia*, which causes Legionnaire's disease, are resistant to damage by the lysosome contents;

(c) some bacteria (e.g. the mainly tick-borne *Rickettsia* species, which cause tropical fevers) can break out of the vacuole in which they were engulfed, into the safety of the macrophage's cytoplasm.

5.2.2 Viral escape strategies

Unlike most bacteria, viruses cannot proliferate outside the cells of their host, so many of the strategies in the list above would be of no use to them. But viruses have evolved a few important tricks of their own; two of the most fascinating are known as **antigenic drift** and **antigenic shift**. In antigenic *drift*, point mutations (single base changes) occur sporadically in the genes coding for immunogenic glycoproteins on the surface envelope of the virus particle.

☐ What effect will this have on the immune response to that virus?

■ An adaptive response developed against the original envelope antigens may be rendered less effective if the epitopes are slightly altered by mutation. This enables the virus to circulate continuously in the population because *previous* hosts will have developed memory cells with high-affinity receptors for the *previous* epitopes, but they are unprotected against the *new* epitopes.

The influenza virus is the most well-known example of a virus that is continually drifting its surface antigens, and there is evidence that the human immunodeficiency virus (HIV) also has this capacity. The influenza virus is also capable of the far more dangerous antigenic *shift*, in which the surface antigens are completely altered by a combination of the genomes from two different strains of influenza virus. This is possible when a single cell is infected simultaneously with both strains. People infected with a totally new strain have no pre-existing immunity and no vaccines exist to protect them. Antigenic shift accounts for the influenza epidemics of the past, including the pandemic of 1919 which killed more than 20 million people world-wide.

The influenza virus and the viruses that cause the common cold have very short incubation times and proliferate in the mucous membranes close to their point of entry into the body. This affords them some protection from immune attack. Viruses that have long incubation periods or that have to travel long distances in the bloodstream to reach their proliferation site are, as a general rule, less successful evaders of the immune response. HIV is the most dangerous exception.

5.2.3 Parasite escape strategies

Unicellular and multicellular parasites have extremely diverse structures and life cycles and display a wide range of escape strategies, some of which have also been evolved by some strains of bacteria and viruses. Parasitic protozoa, such as those causing Chagas disease and sleeping sickness (*Trypanosoma* species), tropical sores (*Leishmania* species), and malaria (*Plasmodium* species), are able to survive inside macrophages and other phagocytic cells by using the mechanisms described in Section 5.2.1 for bacteria (point 6 in the list). Trypanosomes and plasmodia also display antigenic drift, but the surface antigens of each organism are programmed to drift while it is inside the host, so that they remain 'one jump ahead' of the host response. This presents a huge problem for vaccine development.

A few species of highly successful multicellular parasites have also evolved the ability to disguise themselves as the cells of their host (an escape mechanism not seen in pathogenic microbes). For example, *Ascaris lumbricoides* (the most common roundworm infecting the gut) has epitopes on its surface that closely resemble human collagen. The various species of *Schistosoma* (flukes that cause schistosomiasis) go one step further by coating themselves with glycoproteins, MHC molecules and antibodies 'stolen' from their host.

☐ A completely different strategy has been adopted by certain species of worm, which can activate *all* the nearby clones of B cells that produce IgE. At first glance this seems like suicide! How does it protect the worm?

■ If all clones are activated, then the area will be flooded with IgE molecules with numerous different antigen specificities, just a few of which will recognise epitopes on the surface of the worm. Local mast cells will become saturated with all these IgE molecules, which dilutes the number of mast cells with bound IgE that can recognise worm antigens.

The final mechanism that we will mention is the ability of some trypanosomes to secrete substances with a generalised suppressive effect on the immune response. The precise mechanisms are not yet understood, but in infected people suppressor T cells are certainly activated far above the normal level. It has also been shown that trypanosomes inhibit the expression of interleukin-2 receptors on helper T cells.

Summary of Chapter 5

1 The innate and adaptive immune responses enhance and regulate each other; collaboration results in a more effective response than either can achieve alone.

2 Variations exist in the relative contribution of innate and adaptive mechanisms to protecting specific tissues, membranes and circulatory systems from infection, and in the relative effectiveness of specific mechanisms against different pathogens and parasites.

3 A dynamic balance exists between the evolution of improved immune responses in the hosts of pathogens and parasites, and improved escape strategies by infectious organisms; escape cannot be so successful that hosts are destroyed before the infection can be passed on.

4 The evolutionary balance breaks down when a host population is infected by a pathogen that has never been encountered before; when a host is infected by a pathogen that evolved in a different species; when the immune system is suppressed by, for example, infection or malnutrition; or when successful escape strategies are evolved by an infectious organism.

5 Pathogen and parasite escape strategies include structures that inhibit phagocytosis; toxins and enzymes that inhibit or divert host response mechanisms; the ability to survive inside phagocytes; antigenic drift and shift; disguise with host molecules; polyclonal activation of B cells; and immunosuppression.

Now attempt SAQs 19–21, which relate to this Chapter.

CHAPTER 6
ANTIGENS

In this Chapter we look in more detail at antigens and discuss what makes a particular cluster of residues *immunogenic* (i.e. capable of eliciting an adaptive immune response). We aim to give you a few ground rules about immunogenicity, and we discuss the factors affecting the affinity of an epitope for the corresponding binding site on an antibody molecule or T cell receptor. We also discuss cross-reacting antigens and the difference between antigens recognised by B cells and those recognised by T cells.

6.1 General features of antigens

Naturally occurring antigens are extremely diverse. Cell-bound proteins form the largest single group, but many polysaccharide antigens have been identified, and some lipids and even nucleic acids are immunogenic if presented to the right species in the right way. Small organic and inorganic haptens may also act as antigens if they become bound to a carrier protein in the body: penicillin and nickel are two such haptens that can provoke an immune response if they bind to body proteins.

6.1.1 Size

One feature that all immunogenic molecules have in common is a minimum *size*. A relative molecular mass of least M_r 1 000 is required before the immune system will respond to an antigen. However, once an immune response has generated specific antibodies or activated T cells with the correct receptors, these recognition molecules will bind to an epitope of only a few residues in size (e.g. to a hapten without a carrier). Epitopes range in size from a minimum of about five amino acid residues (or sugar units) if they are arranged in a linear sequence, to three or even four times that number if the amino acid side chains are packed together by coiling of the polypeptide.

6.1.2 Structure

Protein antigens have been studied far more extensively than other classes of immunogenic macromolecule. Although B cell clones that recognise non-protein antigens exist, all the T cell clones characterised so far have receptors for proteins. It therefore seems possible that non-protein antigens are T cell-*independent*. The ability of certain carbohydrates and lipids to activate a clone of B cells without T cell help may be a function of their molecular structure. Many polysaccharide and lipid antigens are polymers with repeating sequences that enable adjacent sIg molecules on the B cell to be cross-linked by the antigen (recall Figure 3.6), triggering B cell activation. Proteins are usually considered to be far more varied in their primary and higher-order structure than are polysaccharides and lipids, although the short oligosaccharide chains on glycoproteins and glycolipids can be extremely varied, and are often highly immunogenic.

Like antibodies, antigens are described as having a certain *valency*, which relates to the number of epitopes on the antigen. Naturally occurring antigens are almost always *multivalent*, i.e. they have several structurally different epitopes on the same molecule, and each of these epitopes may occur more than once. Figure 6.1 shows a hypothetical globular protein, with a number of different epitopes formed by *linear* sequences of residues, or *assembled* from residues brought together in space from different parts of the polypeptide chain. Epitopes on the surface and in the interior of the antigen can be recognised by both B cells and T cells (i.e. both have complementary receptors), but the *internal* epitopes are responded to mainly by T cells. The reason for this will become clear in a later part of this Chapter; for the moment, you should note that B cells and T cells generally have receptors for different epitopes.

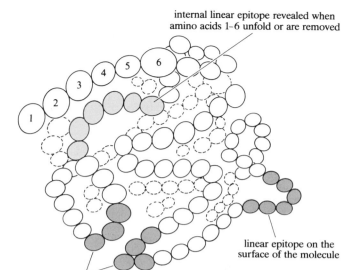

internal linear epitope revealed when amino acids 1–6 unfold or are removed

linear epitope on the surface of the molecule

assembled epitope involving two separate segments of the polypeptide chain

FIGURE 6.1 The epitopes of protein antigens may be on the surface of the molecule or internal to the folding of the polypeptide chain. They may be composed of linear sequences of residues, or assembled from residues from distant parts of the chain and held in a particular conformation by non-covalent interactions.

The structural features of epitopes shown schematically in Figure 6.1 can be found in sperm-whale myoglobin, an oxygen-carrying protein in the muscles of whales. Figure 6.2 shows the known epitopes of sperm-whale myoglobin that are recognised by a particular strain of inbred mouse (the epitopes vary slightly depending on the species or strain of the responder animal). Notice that there is some overlap of residues involved in at least one B cell epitope and one T cell epitope on the surface of the molecule.

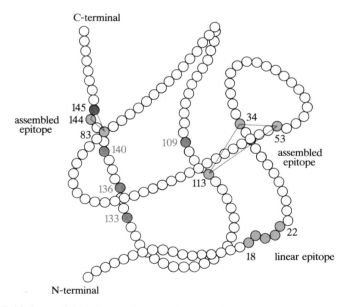

C-terminal

145
assembled   144
epitope
83

140

109

34

53
assembled
epitope

136

113

133

22

18   linear epitope

N-terminal

FIGURE 6.2 Some of the epitopes of sperm whale myoglobin. The amino acid positions are numbered from the N-terminal of the polypeptide chain; residues in epitopes recognised by B cells are shown in grey and those in epitopes recognised by T cells are shown in red. Residues at positions 18 to 22 form a linear epitope that is recognised by a single clone of B cells. Two assembled epitopes, each recognised by a single B cell clone, have also been identified, one incorporating residues at positions 34, 53 and 113, and the other incorporating residues at positions 83, 144 and 145. The residue at position 145 is lysine, and it also forms part of an epitope consisting of residues 133, 136, 140 and 145, which is recognised by a clone of T cells. Residue 109 is glutamic acid and this seems to be involved in another T cell epitope.

6.1.3 'Foreignness'

There is nothing special about the residues that occur in the epitopes of protein antigens in the sense that any of the twenty amino acids can contribute to an epitope. What is important is that the three-dimensional arrangement of the residues in the epitope gives a *shape and charge profile* not normally found on the body cells of the responder organism, or on the macromolecules synthesised by that organism. In other words, epitopes display the property of *'foreignness'*, or difference from self.

But 'foreignness' is a relative concept. The epitopes on a bacterial toxin that are recognised as foreign by (say) a mouse may not appear foreign to a human, and vice versa; or, put more precisely, mice and humans have antigen receptors of different shapes that bind to different parts of the antigen. Moreover, each individual mouse or human has different MHC molecules. This means that the epitopes that are recognised by the T cells of one individual differ from those recognised by another. What appears foreign to you may look like self to me! Thus, in general, there is nothing intrinsically 'foreign' about particular amino acid residues (unlike certain polysaccharides, for example the peptidoglycans, whose component sugars occur only in bacterial cell walls; see Chapter 2); nor is there anything remarkable about those areas of antigens for which no receptors exist in the receptor library of an individual.

6.1.4 Charged and hydrophobic residues

Although all amino acids can contribute to a protein epitope, some residues occur more frequently than others. Residues whose side chains carry a charge (e.g. lysine and glutamic acid) or that enter into hydrophobic interactions (e.g. alanine, valine, leucine and tyrosine) are particularly common in epitopes. For example, the T cell epitope shown in Figure 6.2 consists of lysine residues at positions 133, 140 and 145, with glutamic acid at position 136.

☐   Can you think of a reason for this preponderance of charged and hydrophobic residues in epitopes? (Hint: think of what holds an epitope in the binding site of an antibody molecule or T cell receptor.)

■   The bonding between an epitope and the corresponding antibody or T cell receptor binding site is non-covalent, i.e. it is a combination of *ionic*, *hydrophobic* and *hydrogen bonding*. Thus, charged and hydrophobic residues are essential to antigen binding.

It has been estimated that about half of the binding force between an antigen and the antibody or T cell binding site is due to hydrophobic bonds, which are highly dependent on distance, i.e. they become stronger the closer the opposing residues approach each other. Thus, the 'fit' between the conformation and charge profile of the epitope and that of the corresponding binding site affects the strength of binding between the two. A good fit allows a closer proximity between opposing residues and hence a stronger binding force. The binding force is known as the *affinity* between the epitope and the binding site, and we discuss its estimation for known combinations of antigen and antibody in Section 6.2.1.

The identity of the residues involved in an epitope is often, but not always, critical to antigen recognition. Substitution of one residue for another *may* have no effect whatever on binding by antibody molecules or T cell receptors, or it may abolish binding altogether, or at least reduce the affinity of the epitope for the binding site. The effect depends on the residues involved in the substitution. Obviously, the most influential substitutions involve changes in the charge or hydrophobic profile of the epitope. Even substitutions of residues *outside* the epitope can alter affinity, because a conformational change elsewhere may be relayed to the epitope.

6.1.5 Flexibility

Before we look at affinity measurement in more detail, another feature of antigens that must be considered is the *flexibility of bond angles* between adjacent residues in the epitope and, particularly, in the side chains of residues contributing to the epitope. There is still some uncertainty about the importance of this feature, but several experiments have shown that local mobility of the side chains of certain residues allows the epitope to take up the 'best fit' conformation when in contact with the binding site. This improves the affinity between the epitope and binding site.

6.2 Antigen–antibody interactions

Interactions between antigens and antibodies have been far more extensively studied than the interaction between antigens and T cell receptors. (Remember that the T cell antigen receptor was only sequenced in 1984, and its higher-order structure will be very difficult to determine by crystallographic studies because of its size and complexity.) In addition, it is much easier to estimate the strength of antigen binding when the receptor molecule is 'free', like an antibody, than when it is attached to a cell membrane. The discussion that follows is therefore devoted exclusively to interactions between antigens and antibodies in solution, as might be expected to occur in body fluids.

6.2.1 Affinity measurement

The simplest way to determine the affinity between an antigen and the corresponding binding sites of an antibody molecule is to measure the interaction of a *monovalent* hapten with *divalent* antibodies raised against it. A monovalent hapten has a single epitope on its surface and therefore can bind only a single molecule of antibody. (Note that the antibody can bind two *separate* molecules of hapten, but it cannot cross-link them because each has only one epitope.) When an antibody binds to a complementary antigen the resulting assembly is referred to as an **immune complex**. A complex consisting of a monovalent hapten and its complementary antibody dissociates at a rate that depends on the *affinity* between the epitope and the antigen binding site of the antibody. This dissociation can be expressed by the equation

$$Ab + Hp \rightleftharpoons Ab.Hp \tag{6.1}$$

where Ab is free antibody, Hp is free hapten and Ab.Hp is the immune complex. If the antibody has a very *high* affinity for the hapten, then the equilibrium for this reaction will lie well to the *right*.

The **affinity constant** (K) is given by the equation

$$K = \frac{[Ab.Hp]}{[Ab][Hp]} \tag{6.2}$$

For *high* affinity antibody–hapten complexes,

$$K = \frac{1}{[Hp_{1/2}]} \tag{6.3}$$

at the point where *half* the antibody binding sites are bound to hapten.

This relationship becomes clearer when you understand the method by which the affinity constant is estimated experimentally. The technique is known as **equilibrium dialysis**. A perspex chamber is used in which two compartments are separated by a semi-permeable membrane (Figure 6.3). The membrane allows the free diffusion of hapten molecules but prevents the passage of the much larger antibody molecules.

☐   What would you expect to occur in the two compartments as time passes?

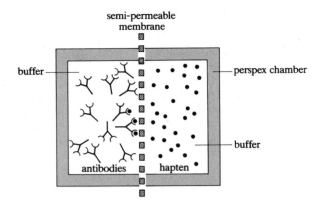

FIGURE 6.3 Apparatus for estimating the affinity between a monovalent hapten and a divalent antibody. The membrane allows diffusion of the hapten molecules but not the antibody molecules.

■ Hapten molecules will diffuse into the compartment containing antibodies and will combine with, and dissociate from, the antibodies. The rate of combination and dissociation will depend on the affinity between the hapten and antigen. At equilibrium, the concentration of *free* hapten in both compartments will be equal.

☐ Suppose that an assay method exists that can measure the total concentration of hapten in either compartment. How could this be used to estimate the amount of *bound* hapten at equilibrium?

■ Measure the concentration of hapten in each compartment. Subtract the concentration of hapten in the hapten-only compartment from the total concentration of free and bound hapten in the compartment that contains the antibodies. The result is the concentration of haptens bound to antibody binding sites at equilibrium.

The concentration of bound haptens at equilibrium will depend not only on the *affinity* of the antibodies for the hapten, but also on the *concentration* of hapten molecules in the equilibrium dialysis chamber. If the concentration of hapten bound to antibodies is plotted for a range of initial hapten concentrations, the graph will take the form shown in Figure 6.4. (This is similar to the estimation of affinity (K_M) between enzymes and their substrates, where the ligand is substrate not hapten, and the plot measures enzyme activity rather than hapten binding; both plots flatten off as the respective binding sites become saturated with bound hapten or substrate.)

The *maximal* concentration of bound hapten also depends on the concentration of *antibodies* present in the dialysis chamber, as well as on their affinity for the hapten. But different samples of antibodies raised against the hapten (e.g. from different individuals, or taken on different days from the same individual) will be at different antibody concentrations, so how can they be compared on the basis of their affinity alone? The problem is solved by estimating the concentration of hapten required for *half* the maximal binding, i.e. the hapten concentration at which *half* the binding sites of the antibodies are filled. At this hapten concentration

$$[Ab.Hp] = \frac{[Ab]}{2} \qquad (6.4)$$

and the affinity constant for a given hapten–antibody interaction is given by

$$K = \frac{1}{[Hp_{1/2}]} \qquad (6.3, \text{ shown earlier})$$

Note from equation 6.3 that the *higher* the affinity of the antibodies for the hapten, the *lower* the concentration of hapten required to occupy half the antibody binding sites, and the *higher* the value of K. The range of affinities for different combinations of haptens and antibodies is quite large, but hapten concentrations of

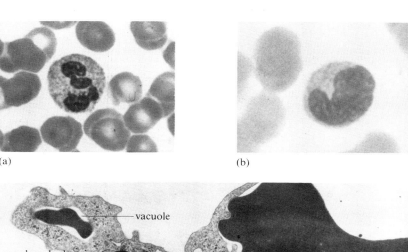

(a)

(b)

PLATE 2.1 Stained blood cells viewed through a light microscope. (a) A neutrophil surrounded by red blood cells; note the many-lobed nucleus. (b) A blood macrophage with characteristic horseshoe or kidney-shaped nucleus; tissue macrophages are even larger and have more cytoplasm around the nucleus (see Plate 2.2a).

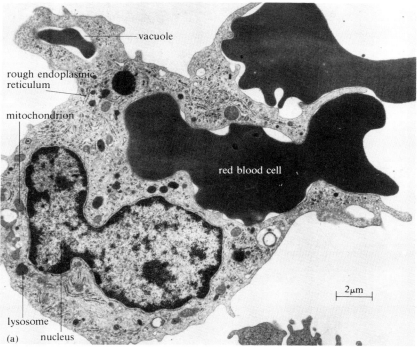

vacuole

rough endoplasmic reticulum

mitochondrion

red blood cell

lysosome

(a)   nucleus

2 μm

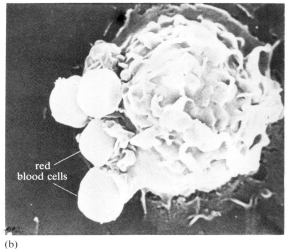

red blood cells

(b)

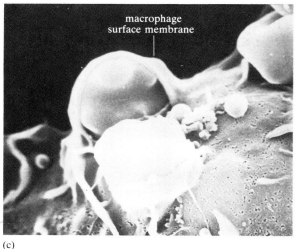

macrophage surface membrane

(c)

PLATE 2.2 (a) An electronmicrograph of a tissue macrophage engulfing red blood cells that were experimentally coated with antigen. Note the shape of the nucleus, the many darkly-stained granules in the cytoplasm and the large size of the cell (about 20 μm in diameter). (b) Scanning electronmicrograph of a macrophage adhering to several red blood cells (magnified about 5 000 times). (c) Close-up of the macrophage surface membrane beginning to enclose the red cell as phagocytosis begins (magnified about 10 000 times).

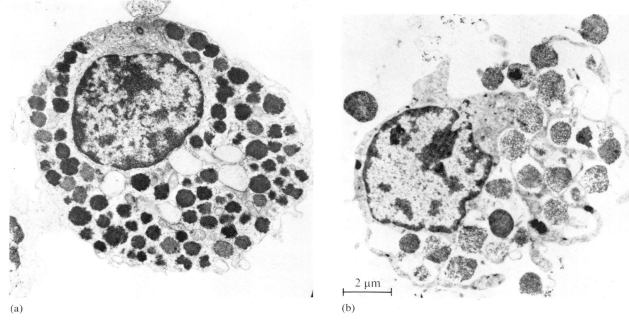

(a)   (b)

PLATE 2.3 (a) Electronmicrograph of a mast cell with many conspicuous, darkly-stained granules in the cytoplasm, which contain chemically active molecules involved in the inflammatory reaction. (b) A mast cell degranulating, i.e. expelling the granules more or less simultaneously through the cell membrane. Despite the extensive disruption of the membrane the cell is not destroyed, but recovers to make new granules. The granules were originally thought to have been imported into the cell by phagocytosis—a misconception which gave rise to the name 'mast cell', from the German word 'Mast' meaning a fattening feed.

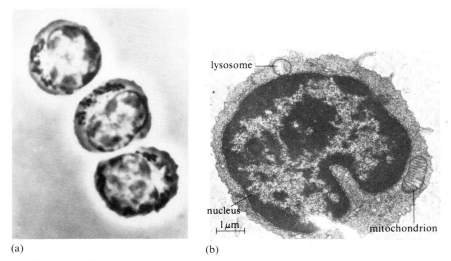

(a)   (b)

PLATE 3.1 Small lymphocytes viewed under (a) a phase-contrast microscope, magnified about 6 000 times, and (b) an electron microscope, magnified about 8 000 times. Note the sparse cytoplasm and organelles, characteristic of small lymphocytes *prior* to contact with the appropriate antigen.

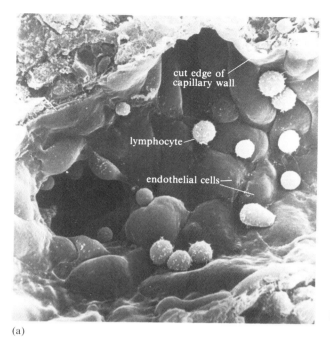

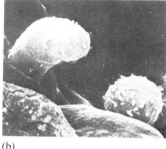

(a)   (b)

PLATE 3.2 (a) Scanning electronmicrograph showing lymphocytes inside a high endothelial venule (the finest venous capillaries passing through lymph nodes). Note the cobblestone appearance of the endothelial cells (magnified about 1 000 times). (b) Close-up view of a lymphocyte starting its journey through the wall of the venule into the lymph node beyond. The endothelial cells will allow only lymphocytes to squeeze past them, and hence lymphocytes are the only white cell that can leave the bloodstream and enter the lymphatic circulation by this route (magnified about 5 000 times).

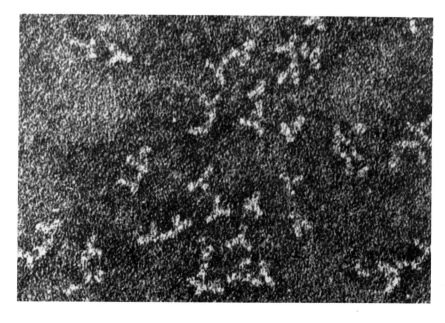

PLATE 4.1 Electronmicrograph of human IgA monomers and dimers, magnified 1.6 million times. The dimers appear to be monomers linked end-to-end at the C-terminal end of the heavy chains, and there is limited flexibility at the junction point.

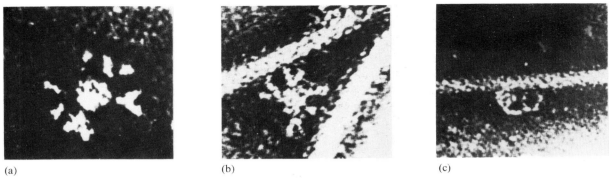

(a)   (b)   (c)

PLATE 4.2 Electronmicrograph of IgM pentamers, magnified about 5 million times. The 'star' formation is shown in (a), where the pentamer is not bound to antigen, and in (b), where it is cross-linking two bacterial flagellae. (c) shows the pentamer in the 'crab' formation with the monomers bent at the hinge to allow maximum contact between the antigen binding sites and, in this case, a bacterial flagellum.

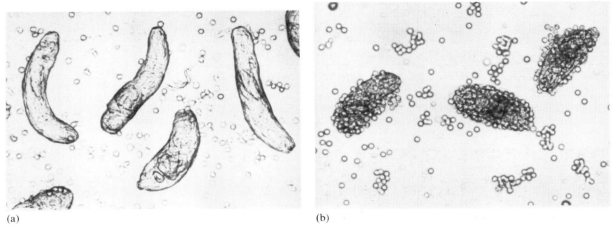

(a)   (b)

PLATE 5.1 Experimental demonstration of antibody-dependent cell-mediated cytotoxicity (ADCC; described in Sections 2.2.2 and 3.2.4) directed against the larvae of *Schistosoma mansonii*, a parasite that infests about 20 million people in Third World countries. (a) The larvae are incubated with neutrophils in an antibody-free culture medium, but very little cytotoxic activity is directed against the parasites. (b) When appropriate antibodies are added, they bind to the schistosomules and the neutrophils bind to the antibodies; the neutrophils are activated to externalise their toxic and pore-forming chemicals, and the larvae are quickly destroyed.

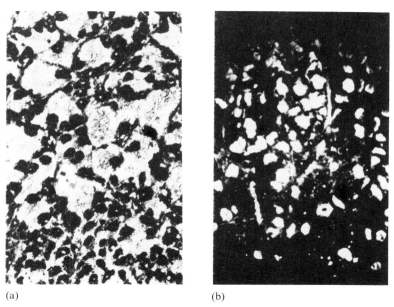

(a)   (b)

PLATE 8.1 Parietal cells from the stomach wall of a patient who produces autoantibodies that have binding sites for epitopes on these cells. The autoantibodies are made visible by (a) peroxidase-linked second antibodies, which bind to the autoantibodies and are then reacted with a suitable substrate to give a black colour; and (b) fluorescein-linked second antibodies, which bind to the autoantibodies and can then be viewed under ultraviolet light in a fluorescence microscope.

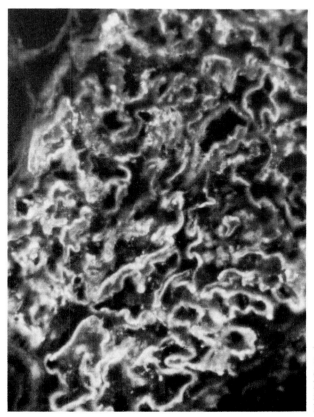

PLATE 10.1 Autoantibodies bound to the basement membrane of kidney glomeruli and made visible by staining with fluorescein-linked second antibodies. This linear pattern of immunofluorescence is typical of the autoimmune condition known as Goodpasture's syndrome (see Table 10.1).

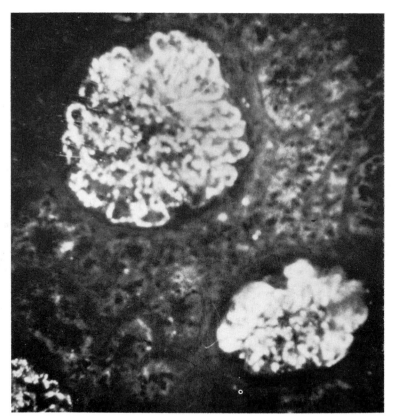

PLATE 10.2 Immune complexes deposited in the kidneys of a person with systemic lupus erythematosus (see Figures 10.5 and 10.9), a condition in which autoantibodies bind to soluble antigens from the person's tissues, particularly to DNA and RNA molecules. The immune complexes have been made visible by immunofluorescence, as in Plate 10.1.

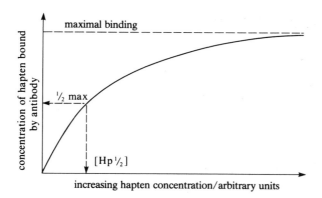

FIGURE 6.4 Estimation of the concentration of a monovalent hapten required to fill half the binding sites of an antibody preparation. Maximal binding is determined for a range of increasing hapten concentrations using the apparatus shown in Figure 6.3, and the results are plotted as a graph. The hapten concentration $[Hp_{1/2}]$ that gives half-maximal binding (1/2 max) can then be read from the graph.

between 10^{-4} mol l^{-1} and as low as 10^{-10} mol l^{-1} have been measured experimentally as giving half-maximal binding to their corresponding antibodies. When concentrations as low as this can fill half the binding sites of the antibody molecules, you can see just how high the affinity between the hapten and the antibody must be. The affinity between most haptens and their complementary antibodies is several orders of magnitude greater than the affinity between even the highest affinity enzyme–substrate combinations.

6.2.2 Avidity

In life, antigens are a lot more complex than the monovalent haptens that we have been discussing here. A virus particle, for example, or a molecule of bacterial toxin, may be multivalent for the same epitope, and/or have dozens of entirely different epitopes on its surface and a few more hidden away in its internal structure. The forces governing the affinity of monovalent haptens and antibodies apply equally to more complex antigen–antibody pairings, but in practice the estimation of the affinity between a complex antigen and a sample of antibodies is made using Fab antibody fragments rather than whole antibody molecules.

☐ Can you deduce why?

■ Complex antigens are often multivalent, i.e. they have many identical epitopes on their surface. Whole antibody molecules have at least two binding sites, so they can cross-link similar or identical epitopes on the same or even on different antigen molecules, and this interferes with the affinity estimation (you will see why in a moment). This problem is overcome by using detached Fab regions. Each Fab fragment is monovalent, i.e. it has a single binding site, so it can bind to a single epitope and affinity estimation will not be affected by cross-linking.

Naturally occurring antigens generally have many entirely different epitopes on their surface and as a result will activate many different clones of B cells, each secreting antibodies with binding sites for one of the epitopes. The serum containing a mixed sample of antibodies generated in response to a complex multivalent antigen is known collectively as an **antiserum**. Antisera also contain antibodies that bind to the *same* epitope, but with a range of affinities. This is because several B cell clones may have receptors with a range of affinities for the same epitope. So, an antiserum contains many different *species* of antibody, each one distinguished from the others by its epitope specificity and affinity. You might expect the *collective* affinity of the antiserum for the complex antigen to be an *average* of the different affinities of each species of antibody in the antiserum. But a further complication exists.

The *functional* (actual) affinity of an antiserum for a given multivalent antigen is known as the **avidity** of the antiserum. In practice, the avidity of an antiserum for a complex antigen is always many times *greater* than the sum of the affinities of each antibody species for each epitope. In fact, the affinity constant K for an antiserum in contact with a complex antigen is obtained by *multiplying* the contributing individual affinities. The reason why avidity exceeds individual affinity by so much is shown in Figure 6.5.

The multiplying effect results from the multiple cross-linking of epitopes on adjacent antigen molecules (Figure 6.5a) by antibodies with different epitope specificities. Each specificity has a different affinity for its epitope and so will dissociate from it and reassociate with it at a characteristic rate. This is a dynamic situation, with antibodies dissociating from the bound state and reassociating continually. When one antibody bridge spontaneously dissociates (Figure 6.5b), other bridges remain, at least for a time. These hold the molecules of antigen together for long enough to allow the dissociated antibody to reassociate and re-form an antibody bridge far more quickly than it could do if it were the sole cross-link. Without the bridging by other antibodies, the two molecules of antigen would drift apart when the antibody with the lowest affinity dissociated from its epitope. This is analogous to a man hanging on to a cliff with both hands and occasionally relaxing his grip with one or other hand—he can still hang on. But if he had been holding on with only one hand to start with, and then he relaxed his grip…!

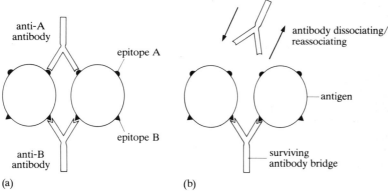

(a) (b)

FIGURE 6.5 The avidity of an antiserum for a multivalent antigen is greater than the sum of the individual contributing affinities because the binding energy of the interaction between antibodies with different epitope specificities is multiplied (a) by multiple cross-linking of adjacent antigen molecules, and (b) by surviving antibody bridges holding the antigens together during the period in which other antibody bridges dissociate and reassociate.

☐ Would you expect the avidity of an antiserum with a high concentration of IgM antibodies to be higher or lower than the avidity of an IgG antiserum against the same antigen?

■ It would be higher because the potential for cross-linking adjacent antigens is much greater for IgM (with its ten binding sites) than for IgG (with only two).

To some extent, this magnification of avidity of IgM antisera compensates for the lower *individual* affinity of each IgM binding site for the epitope. (You may recall from Chapter 4 that affinity maturation accompanies the class switch from IgM to IgG, which occurs during the generation of memory cells in the primary response.)

6.2.3 Cross-reacting antigens

Many times in this Book we have referred to an antibody molecule as having a binding site for a *specific* epitope. But just how exclusive is the interaction between an antibody and the epitope that provoked its synthesis? In practice, structurally related but different epitopes may be bound by antibody molecules with binding sites that precisely fit only one of them. These epitopes are described as *cross-*

reacting with the antibody. As you would expect, the affinity of the antibody for a range of similar epitopes is *lower* than its affinity for the 'best fit' epitope. Table 6.1 illustrates the reduction in affinity of an antibody preparation raised against hapten X (Figure 6.6) when mixed with five related haptens. Notice that there is a 50-fold decrease in affinity for hapten 2 compared with the affinity for hapten 1; their chemical structure is identical, but hapten 2 is a partial mirror image of hapten 1.

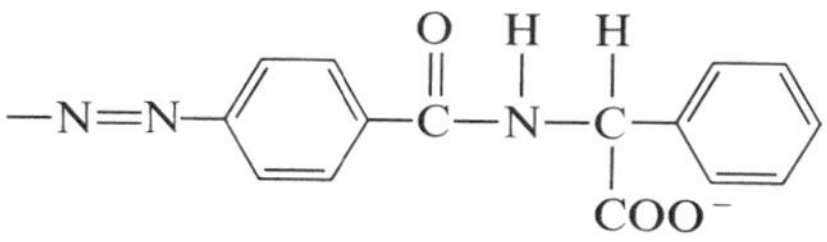

FIGURE 6.6 Hapten X

TABLE 6.1 Affinity of antibodies raised against hapten X when tested against related haptens 1 to 5

Test hapten	Average affinity $K_A/l \, mmol^{-1}$
(1)	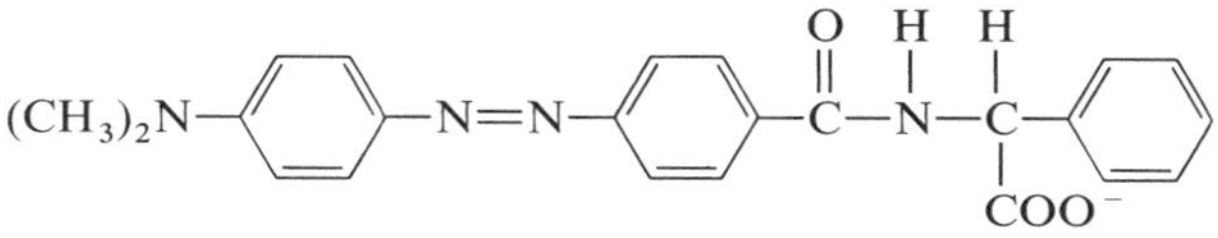 500
(2)	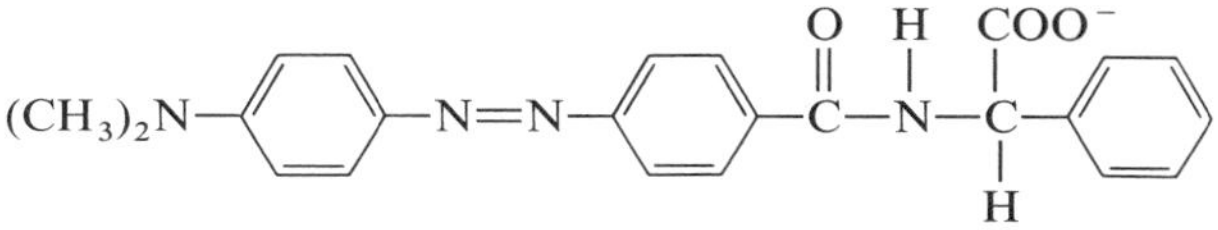 10
(3)	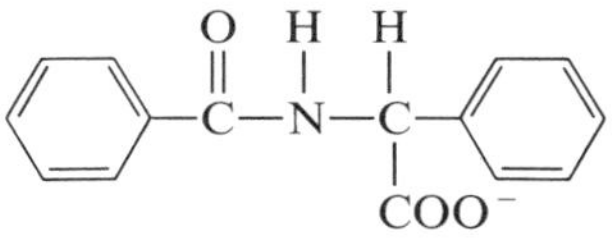 100
(4)	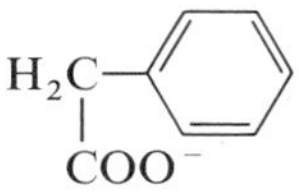 1.5
(5)	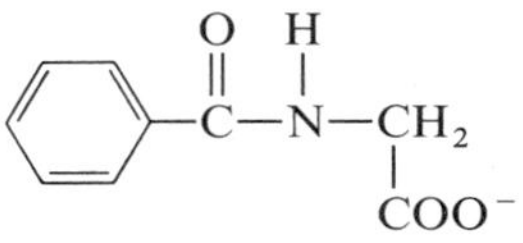 0.1

Cross-reaction between antibody molecules with a particular specificity and a range of closely related epitopes may help to extend immune protection to closely related strains of pathogen. Once a person has recovered from an infection with one strain, then other strains with similar epitopes may elicit a secondary immune response even when they are encountered for the first time (Figure 6.7a). However, there is another form of cross-reactivity which is probably more important in extending immunity in life. Although each individual strain of pathogen has some *unique* epitopes in its structure, closely related strains also share *identical* epitopes (Figure 6.6b). Thus, some of the antibody specificities in an antiserum raised against (say) a particular strain of virus will also recognise identical epitopes on a related virus strain. This is precisely the type of cross-reactivity that Edward Jenner exploited in 1796 when he inoculated a boy with cowpox virus and later demonstrated that the child was immune to the virus that causes smallpox.

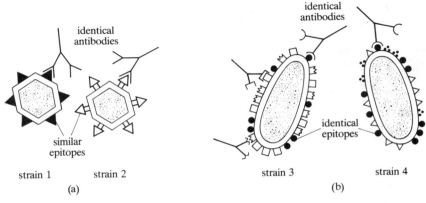

identical
antibodies

identical
antibodies

similar
epitopes

identical
epitopes

strain 1   strain 2

strain 3   strain 4

(a)   (b)

FIGURE 6.7 Cross-reacting antigens. (a) Antibodies raised against the epitopes of strain 1 also bind to the structurally similar epitopes of strain 2, but with a lower affinity. Recovery from infection with strain 1 gives some protection against infection with strain 2. (b) Strains 3 and 4 share at least one identical epitope, although their other epitopes are unique to each strain. Infection with strain 3 generates antibodies against all its epitopes, including the shared epitope; this confers some protection against infection with strain 4.

6.3   B cell and T cell epitopes

Earlier in this Chapter we noted in passing that although some of the epitopes recognised by B cells and T cells overlap, other epitopes are recognised only by B cells *or* T cells. This is another example of 'division of labour' in the immune response. B cells seem to respond mainly to epitopes on the surface of antigens, infectious cells or virus particles. T cells, by contrast, can also recognise epitopes that are buried inside globular proteins or that are part of the internal structure of pathogens and parasites. This is illustrated in Figure 6.8, which shows the epitopes on the haemagglutinin molecule of the influenza virus that are recognised by B cells, by T cells and by both.

Another important difference is that T cells can generally still bind to epitopes that have been *separated* from the antigen molecule, whereas most B cells bind only to epitopes on the *intact* (native) antigen. B cells that bound previously to an intact protein antigen generally fail to bind to the *denatured* protein, or to polypeptide *fragments* cleaved from it (there are exceptions to this, but it is a reasonable generalisation). Similarly, antibodies that bound to epitopes on the intact protein generally fail to bind to those epitopes on the denatured or cleaved protein.

☐   Can you explain this phenomenon?

■   The interaction between the epitope and the binding site (whether on secreted antibody molecules or surface-bound immunoglobulin) is dependent on the residues in the epitope taking up a particular conformation in three dimensions. Denaturation or splitting the antigen into polypeptides destroys the tertiary structure of the molecule and hence the conformation of the epitopes. Even linear epitopes may no longer bind to the antibody because their conformation can vary so extensively once the polypeptide containing the epitope is freed from the constraints placed on it by the rest of the molecule.

Although there are exceptions, most T cells still manage to bind to epitopes when the intact protein has been denatured or cleaved, and (unlike B cells) T cells can recognise *internal* (as opposed to surface) epitopes.

☐   Can you explain these differences between antigen recognition by B cells and by T cells? (Hint: think about the T cell's requirement for associative recognition of the epitope plus the appropriate class of MHC molecule.)

■ B cells recognise antigens alone, whereas T cells require antigens to be presented to them on the surface of antigen-presenting cells (APCs) in association with MHC molecules. The B cell's receptor binds to epitopes that are readily accessible on the surface of the intact antigen, whereas the antigens recognised by T cells have first been engulfed by APCs and 'processed' (degraded) before the epitope resurfaces and associates with the MHC molecules. The processing of the antigen in the APC exposes 'hidden' epitopes, which were internal to the structure. But processing also destroys the structural conformation of the antigen, so most T cells must be able to recognise short linear epitopes.

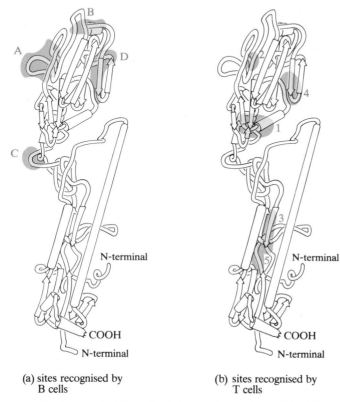

(a) sites recognised by B cells

(b) sites recognised by T cells

FIGURE 6.8 The haemagglutinin molecule is a surface antigen of the influenza strain A virus. (a) The four epitopes (A–D, in red) recognised by B cell clones are all on the *surface* of the molecule and in the 'head' region of the chain. (b) However, four of the five epitopes (in red) recognised by T cells (epitopes 1–3 and 5) are in the *internal* structure of the molecule, and epitopes 3 and 5 are in the less accessible 'tail'. There is overlap between epitope D (a B cell epitope) and epitope 4 (a T cell epitope).

6.4 Allogeneic and xenogeneic antigens

So far in this Chapter we have confined ourselves to discussing antigens that arise from pathogens and parasites, or that result from the 'accidental' combination of small molecules, such as penicillin, with body proteins. We conclude with a brief review of those antigens that appear on the surface of vertebrate cells and that are recognised as foreign if the cells are transplanted into another member of the same species (**allogeneic antigens**) or into a different species (**xenogeneic antigens**). Note that these epitopes are not normally immunogenic in the animal from which they originated.

☐ You already know a great deal about some of the most important allogeneic antigens. What are they?

■ Certain parts of the MHC molecules are allogeneic antigens. These epitopes are the targets for the immune response that results in graft rejection when tissue or organs are transplanted between non-identical individuals of the same species. (They were formerly known as *transplantation* antigens.)

6.4.1 Blood group antigens

Another important category of allogeneic antigens are the **blood group antigens**—a variety of glycoproteins found on the surface membrane of red blood cells. The most important blood group antigens are those by which blood is classified into Group O, A, B or AB, and either Rhesus-positive or Rhesus-negative. The **ABO** (say *ay-bee-oh*) blood group antigens are three structurally related glycoproteins that occur on red cells and free in saliva and seminal fluid. They each have a M_r of about 10^6 and share a common glycoprotein known as *H-substance*. Individuals with Group O blood have H-substance alone on their red cells; the Group A antigen is H-substance joined to *N*-acetylgalactosamine (Figure 6.9a); and the Group B antigen is H-substance linked to D-galactose (Figure 6.9b). Individuals with type AB blood have both the Group A and the Group B antigens on their red cells.

In *theory*, transfusing blood between individuals with different blood group antigens would eventually result in the synthesis of antibodies directed against the antigens that differed from those on the respondent's red cells. However, nature got their first! Everyone with Group A blood produces antibodies directed against the Group B antigen, and Group B individuals produce antibodies directed against the Group A antigen. Group O individuals produce antibodies spontaneously against Group A *and* Group B antigens, and individuals with AB blood don't produce antibodies to *either*. Notice that no-one produces spontaneous antibodies to the Group O antigen. The reason for the apparently spontaneous existence of antibodies against Group A or Group B antigens probably lies in the common occurrence of the immunogenic sugars *N*-acetylgalactosamine and D-galactose in the polysaccharides in bacterial cell walls.

□ Why, do you suppose, does a person with Group A blood produce antibodies to D-galactose (part of the Group B antigen) but not to N-acetylgalactosamine?

■ The antibodies to D-galactose would be formed when the person was exposed to bacteria with D-galactose in their structure, and since these bacteria are so common, everyone will have encountered them at an early age. However, *N*-acetylgalactosamine is part of the Group A antigen and individuals are normally *self-tolerant* (Chapter 1), i.e. an immune response is not normally directed against molecules that occur as part of the individual's own cells or fluids. Thus, even though the person with blood group A will have been exposed many times to bacteria with *N*-acetylgalactosamine in their structure, antibodies against this sugar will not have been produced.

The existence of blood group antigens and antibodies that bind to them necessitates the careful 'typing' of blood group in the donor and the recipient of a blood transfusion. As a general rule, the amount of blood transfused into a patient over time is much less than the blood volume of the patient, so any antibodies in the *transfused* blood are diluted to an extent that renders them harmless to the recipient. However, if the recipient has pre-existing antibodies to the antigens on the *donated* red cells a far more serious situation results.

□ The antibodies against the blood group antigens are nearly all of the IgM class. Can you predict what would happen if a patient were transfused with red cells to which he or she had IgM antibodies?

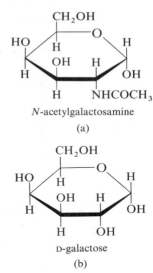

N-acetylgalactosamine

(a)

D-galactose

(b)

FIGURE 6.9 Terminal parts of the blood group antigens found on (a) Group A red cells, and (b) Group B red cells. These sugars are also common in bacterial cell walls.

■ IgM pentamers are able to cross-link antigens very proficiently, so *agglutination* of the transfused red cells occurs and clumps of cells can block capillaries, especially in the kidneys. Bound IgM is also the most powerful activator of the complement cascade, so the donated red cells would be lysed and inflammatory reactions set off throughout the vascular system. Transfusion reactions can result in death of the patient, usually from kidney failure.

☐ Must transfusions of whole blood (as opposed to cell-free serum) be restricted to donors and recipients of the *same* blood group?

■ No. Provided that the volume of the transfusion is not massive, then whole Group O blood can be transfused into patients of *any* blood group. This is because the recipient will not have antibodies to the Group O antigen since H-substance is found on everyone's red cells, and the anti-A and anti-B antibodies in the transfusion are diluted by the patient's blood. (Group O individuals are thus sometimes referred to as *universal donors*.)

The **Rhesus antigen** (also known as the D-antigen) is another blood group antigen that is either present (Rh+) or absent (Rh−) from a person's red cells. Its distribution is independent of the ABO antigens, so individuals of any ABO type may be either Rh+ or Rh−. People do not make antibodies spontaneously to the Rhesus antigen, so no harm results from the first transfusion of Rh+ blood cells into a Rh− individual, but the recipient would synthesise antibodies directed against the Rhesus antigen after a time. These antibodies are mainly of the IgG class. A second blood transfusion of the same type as the first would result in the lysis of many of the transfused red cells by complement triggered by bound IgG. This is not nearly as serious a problem as the extensive agglutination of red cells that can result from an ABO mismatch, but it should nevertheless be avoided by Rhesus-matching. Rh− blood can of course be freely transfused into Rh+ recipients.

☐ However, serious problems arise when a Rh− woman becomes pregnant with her *second* (but not her first) Rh+ baby. Can you deduce why?

■ During the first birth some of the baby's Rh+ red cells leak into the mother's bloodstream as the placenta tears away from the wall of the uterus, and she subsequently makes antibodies against the Rhesus antigen. These antibodies are mainly IgG, which is the only class of immunoglobulin that can cross the placenta. During the second pregnancy, these antibodies enter the baby's circulation and destroy its Rh+ red cells.

This results in a serious anaemia in the baby, known as *haemolytic disease of the new-born*. Affected babies appear yellow from the bilirubin in their circulation, which arises from the breakdown of haemoglobin, and they have difficulty obtaining enough oxygen. This condition was often fatal in the past, but has more or less been abolished in western countries by injecting Rh− women with pre-formed anti-Rhesus antibodies at the birth of the first Rh+ baby. These antibodies lead to the rapid destruction of any Rh+ red cells which have leaked from the baby into the mother's bloodstream, thus destroying the Rhesus antigens before they have the opportunity to evoke an immune response in the mother. The injected antibodies are gradually catabolised (the half-life of IgG in serum is about 23 days; see Table 4.1) and so cause no harm if the woman becomes pregnant with a Rh+ baby for the second time.

6.4.2 Tissue-specific antigens

Cells of a particular histological type (for example, nerve cells or liver cells) may have surface-membrane antigens that are unique to that tissue in that species. These antigens are not immunogenic in other individuals of the *same* species (i.e. they are not allogeneic antigens), but they will provoke an immune response if the cells are injected into an animal of another species (i.e. they are xenogeneic antigens). These **tissue-specific antigens** probably act as identifying markers during morphogenesis, enabling cells to interact and orient themselves correctly as tissues and organs form. In certain *autoimmune* diseases (discussed in detail in Chapter 10), an inappropriate immune response arises against a tissue-specific antigen, with serious consequences for the functional integrity of the tissue involved.

6.4.3 Differentiation and embryonic antigens

Molecules that appear briefly on cells during embryonic life, or when mature cells differentiate from their embryonic precursor, may be immunogenic in other members of the same species or in other species. In other words, parts of the structure of these molecules are unique to each individual and are responded to as foreign antigens if they are transferred to another individual. For example, T cells and B cells express certain glycoproteins at characteristic stages during their differentiation, and it is possible to induce an immune response against these molecules in other members of the same species if immature cells from one individual are injected into another. These molecules are, therefore, *simultaneously* surface markers of lymphocyte differentiation in the originating animal and **differentiation antigens** if exposed to other members of the same species (this is a good example of the relativity of 'selfness' and 'foreignness').

Embryonic cells also express certain glycoproteins, which are lost as the cell matures. These molecules can elicit an immune response if presented to the adult immune system, so they are referred to as **embryonic antigens**. They are of particular interest because some of the glycoproteins that occur on the surface of malignant cells have been shown to be structurally very close to them. This finding has contributed to the re-thinking about the nature of malignant transformation that has marked the last decade; cancer cells are no longer considered to be 'foreign' in the way that the cells of pathogens are, but as body cells that have reverted to a more embryonic form. We discuss this further in the last Chapter of this Book.

Summary of Chapter 6

1 Members of any of the four main classes of biological macromolecules (proteins, polysaccharides, lipids and nucleic acids) can be immunogenic if presented in the right way to the immune system. Most of the antigens found on eukaryote cell surfaces are polypeptides or glycoproteins; polysaccharide antigens are common on prokaryote cells.

2 Immunogenic molecules are large (over M_r 1 000), but the epitopes to which antibodies and T cell receptors bind generally consist of only a few amino acid residues or carbohydrate units.

3 Epitopes may be on the surface of the antigen or within its structure. The residues may be in a linear sequence or assembled from distant parts of the polypeptide chain.

4 Epitopes are 'foreign' only in the sense that residues in that precise conformation do not occur in accessible sites on the cells or macromolecules of the responder organism. The epitopes recognised by one individual or species may differ from the epitopes recognised by another.

5 Epitopes contain a high proportion of charged and hydrophobic residues, which contribute to the non-convalent forces binding the epitope to the antibody or T cell receptor.

6 The affinity contant K for the interaction between the epitope and the binding site is a measure of the rate of spontaneous association and dissociation between the two. When K is large, the affinity of the antibody for the antigen is large, and

the number of epitopes required to fill half the binding sites in an antiserum is small. Therefore, antibodies with a high affinity can bind the complementary antigen efficiently even when the antigen concentration is low.

7   The avidity of an antiserum raised against a multivalent antigen greatly exceeds the sum of the contributing affinities of individual antibodies directed against different epitopes. This 'bonus' effect is due to the cross-linking of antigen molecules.

8   Complex multivalent antigens may share structurally related, or even identical, epitopes. Antibodies raised against the epitopes on one such antigen will cross-react (i.e. bind) with any other antigen that has sufficiently similar epitopes. The affinity of the antibodies for the cross-reacting epitopes will be *lower* than their affinity for the originating epitopes, unless the epitopes are identical.

9   B cells and T cells recognise different epitopes. B cells generally recognise epitopes on the surface of intact antigens, but they can respond to certain carbohydrate and lipid antigens for which T cells have no receptors. T cells only recognise protein antigens, and the epitopes are generally short, linear peptides. T cells can bind to denatured or fragmented antigens. This is probably because in life they respond to epitopes that had been internal to the antigen structure and that became exposed only after the antigen had been processed by antigen-presenting cells.

10   Vertebrate cells and macromolecules have epitopes that are immunogenic either in other members of the same species (allogeneic antigens) or in other species (xenogeneic antigens). MHC molecules, blood group antigens, differentiation antigens and embyonic antigens are important allogeneic antigens; tissue-specific antigens are xenogeneic antigens, but autoimmune reactions against them can occur in some diseases.

Now attempt SAQs 22–24, which relate to this Chapter.

CHAPTER 7
APPLICATIONS OF ANTIGEN RECOGNITION

This Chapter is an introduction to some of the most commonly used methods for detecting, quantifying and purifying antigens using antibodies with a known antigen specificity. The antigens of interest to medical, biological or industrial research may be naturally occurring macromolecules in solution or in the structure of an organism or cell, or they may be artificially constructed from small organic or inorganic haptens covalently linked to large protein carriers. Antibodies are themselves antigens when presented correctly to the immune system of an appropriate animal, and several of the techniques described in this Chapter detect antibodies by treating them as antigens. If the antigen is a molecule that is part of the normal structure of a person's cells, or a macromolecule such as a hormone, then the antibodies are termed *autoantibodies* because they are 'anti-self'. Auto-antibodies are involved in inappropriate immune responses directed against the person's own cells or macromolecules (*autoimmune diseases* are discussed in Chapter 10).

We cannot hope to cover all the methods currently used in hospital, academic or commercial laboratories, but the selection discussed here should give you an overview of the *variety* of applications of antigen recognition.

7.1 Producing the antibodies

Antibodies with binding sites for particular epitopes can be used to identify and 'capture' an antigen even when it is in a complex mixture of molecules. Multivalent antibodies can precipitate a soluble antigen out of solution, or agglutinate cells that have the antigen as part of their structure. Antibodies linked to readily detectable molecules or groups (e.g. fluorescent or radioactive compounds) can be used to locate an antigen and quantify it. So the starting point of all the methods for antigen detection is the production of antibodies with binding sites for the antigen of interest.

☐ What properties would the most useful antibodies have?

■ They would have high *specificity* for epitopes on the antigen, i.e. they would not cross-react with similar epitopes on other contaminating antigens; they would have high *affinity* for the epitopes, so that even if the antigen was very dilute or dispersed the antibodies would still bind to a high proportion of the antigen molecules; and they would be highly *concentrated*, so that the largest possible number of binding sites would be available to the antigen.

In practice, of course, it is not always possible or even necessary to meet all three of these criteria when antibodies are produced. If the antigen of interest differs only very slightly from contaminating antigens, then specificity and affinity would be of such importance that antibodies in low concentration might still be adequate for the task, provided that the method of detection chosen was sufficiently sensitive. Conversely, the antibody preparations used to purify antigens in large amounts may not need to be very specific, and high concentration might be the prime consideration. There are other considerations too, which depend on the chosen method for detecting the antigen.

☐ If the method involves precipitating soluble antigens out of solution, or agglutinating antigenic cells, which *class* of antibodies would be the most useful.

■ IgM would be most useful because of its valency (a theoretical maximum of ten binding sites per pentamer, but fewer in practice), which enables multiple cross-linking of identical epitopes on adjacent antigen molecules.

However, the concentration of IgM in serum is not very high (usually below ten per cent of the total immunoglobulin; see Table 4.1), and its binding sites tend to have a relatively low affinity for the epitope compared with those of IgG. The serum concentration of IgG is seven to eight times higher than that of IgM, so it is much easier to obtain high concentrations of IgG antibodies from peripheral blood, especially during the secondary response. But the fact that IgG is *divalent* (has only two binding sites) makes it a rather poor precipitator or agglutinator of antigens. However, most antigens are *multivalent*, so an antiserum usually contains a mixture of IgG antibodies from different clones of B cells, each with binding sites for a *different* epitope on the *same* antigen. The *avidity* of this antibody mixture is greater than the sum of the individual affinities of each antibody specificity because many more cross-links can be formed between adjacent molecules of antigen. Thus, methods that employ precipitation or agglutination as their end-point tend to use *polyclonal antisera*, that is, a mixture of antibodies obtained from the serum of animals injected with the antigen of interest.

7.1.1 Polyclonal antiserum production

When a multivalent antigen is injected into a suitable recipient, the clones of B (and T) cells with receptors for epitopes on that antigen are activated. If several injections of the antigen are given over a period of weeks and then serum is collected, it will contain *polyclonal* antibodies and is described as a **polyclonal antiserum**. The animals in which polyclonal antisera are 'raised' tend to be from the larger species of domestic mammal, such as rabbits, sheep and goats, because relatively large quantities of serum can be obtained without harming the animal. They are kept as far as possible in conditions that are free from specific pathogens, and of course they should not have been injected with other antigens previously. However, the polyclonal antiserum may also contain contaminating antibodies with binding sites for unrelated antigens that the animal has been exposed to in recent life, or more probably to other antigens in the immunising preparation (it is often the case that the antigen used to immunise the animal is itself impure). This is not a problem as long as the contaminating antibodies don't cross-react with the antigen of interest—but what if they do?

☐ Suggest two strategies for separating out the contaminating antibodies using antigens.

■ (a) Remove the *contaminating* antibodies by exposing the antiserum to a panel of irrelevant antigens to which the contaminating antibodies bind, leaving the wanted antibodies unbound in solution.
(b) Remove the *wanted* antibodies by exposing the antiserum to the immunising antigen so that the wanted antibodies are trapped in immune complexes; the unbound contaminating antibodies can then be washed away.

In both methods, the adsorbing antigens are commonly fixed to a solid matrix—usually a chromatography column packed with beads made from sugar polymers, e.g. agarose. The *contaminating* antibodies will be retained in the column if a panel of irrelevant antigens to which they bind is fixed to the matrix, and the *wanted* antibodies will pass through. Conversely, the *wanted* antibodies will be retained in a column to which the immunising antigen has been coupled. The contaminating antibodies are washed out of the column, and then the wanted antibodies are released from the immune complexes by reducing the binding energy between the antibody and antigen (various methods are used to achieve this; for example, high or low pH solutions may be washed through the column, followed by a buffer to restore the pH to neutral and with it the native conformation of the antibody binding sites). This method is known as **immuno-affinity chromatography**.

☐ There are problems with both these methods of purifying antisera (i.e. adsorbing either the contaminating or the wanted antibodies by complexing them with antigens in chromatography columns). Can you suggest what they are?

■ Adsorbing the *contaminating* antibodies requires a suitable panel of antigens that is totally free from the antigen of interest and does not cross-react with it, but such a panel may not exist. (The reason for wanting the specific antibodies in the first place may have been to separate the antigen of interest from a heavily contaminated mixture.) Adsorbing the *wanted* antibodies requires a sufficiently pure preparation of the injected antigen to couple to the column, but again this may not exist.

A further complication of immunoaffinity chromatography is that the method used to release the wanted antibodies from the immune complexes inevitably disrupts or *denatures* the binding sites. Unless the subsequent *renaturation* of the antibodies is complete, their specificity and affinity for the antigen will be reduced. Moreover, the lowest affinity antibodies are released from the column *first* and the highest affinity antibodies *last*—if at all—and these may be precisely the antibodies that are wanted. Neither method is ideal for purifying a polyclonal antiserum so that it contains as many of the wanted antibody molecules with as few contaminants as possible. The method chosen depends partly on the availability of suitable antigens and partly on the desired properties of the emergent antiserum.

☐ There are other difficulties associated with the production of polyclonal antisera, which centre on the use of animals. Aside from the obvious ethical objections, can you suggest any practical problems?

■ There is a limit to how much serum you can obtain from the same animal (or colony) in a single batch. Once the batch is used up you have to start all over again, raising and purifying a new batch, and this usually has a slightly different composition of antigen specificities and affinities from the first.

However, despite the difficulties of production and purification outlined above, polyclonal antisera will always have an important role in methods that detect antigens by precipitation or agglutination because of their ability to form multiple cross-links between antigens. A number of these methods are described in Section 7.3. But first we will look at a technical breakthrough in antibody production in 1975 that solved a number of the standardisation and purification problems associated with polyclonal antisera.

7.1.2 Monoclonal antibody preparation

Antibodies secreted by plasma cells from a single clone are identical in both their antigen specificity and in their affinity for a particular epitope. Among the many clones activated when a complex multivalent antigen is injected into an experimental animal, there is at least one (probably more) with high-affinity receptors for epitopes that are unique to that antigen. The output of these clones would constitute a highly specific 'probe' for a particular antigen if it could be collected in an uncontaminated form—for example, by growing individual clones of activated B cells in isolation in tissue culture. However, prior to 1975 it was impossible to do this in practice because B cells do not survive in tissue culture for more than a week or two.

The immunologists Cesar Milstein and Georges Köhler overcame this problem by fusing antigen-activated B cells with tumour cells derived from malignant B lymphocytes (these tumours are called *myelomas* or *plasmacytomas*). In the correct tissue culture conditions, the tumour cells are immortal—they go on growing by cell division indefinitely—unlike the B cells, which soon die out. The details of the fusion technique are not relevant here, but the fused cells—termed **hybridomas** by Milstein and Köhler—have the desirable properties of both the fusion partners: they secrete antibodies with the same antigen specificity as the parent B cell and they are immortal if properly cared for. The hybridomas are then *cloned*, that is, grown separately in tissue culture so that the progeny of a single hybrid cell are isolated and multiplied, and then screened to identify which clone (or clones) is producing the desired antibodies. Figure 7.1 summarises the main steps in the production of these **monoclonal antibodies** (often abbreviated to **Mabs**).

☐ Monoclonal antibodies have several significant advantages compared with polyclonal antisera, and only one major disadvantage. Can you suggest what these are?

■ The *advantages* are that a pure preparation of antibodies of known specificity and affinity, and of a single immunoglobulin class, can be obtained in unlimited quantities (at least in theory), with no difference between batches and no need to remove contaminating antibodies.

The main *disadvantage* is that monoclonal antibodies are rather poor at precipitating or agglutinating soluble or cellular antigens because they bind to only one epitope shape, which may occur only once on the antigen. (However, even this problem can be overcome by mixing several Mabs, each with binding sites for a different epitope on the same antigen.)

The other drawbacks of monoclonal antibody production are that it is labour intensive and depends to some extent on luck. A single mouse spleen may yield

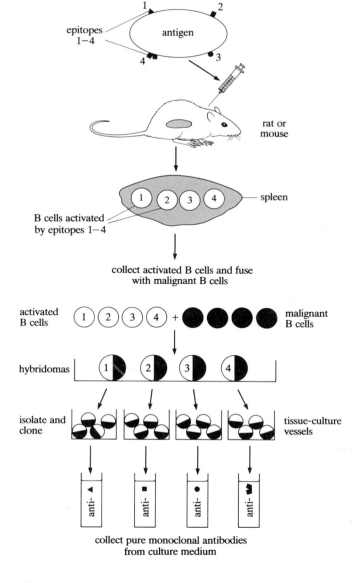

FIGURE 7.1 The main stages in the preparation of four different monoclonal antibodies (Mabs), each with binding sites for a different epitope on the injected antigen.

several million B cells, but the hybridising technique may not succeed in fusing the few that are secreting the antibodies of choice. The successful hybridomas must be screened repeatedly to weed out the uninteresting ones, and the desired clones have to be fed and regularly subdivided as they outgrow their container. Some laboratories inject hybridomas into mice, which act as hosts for the clone, but harvesting Mabs grown in this way raises some of the problems of contaminating antibodies that we discussed earlier in relation to polyclonal antisera. But the advantage of having a standardised source of pure monospecific antibodies that reliably identify a precise epitope outweighs these technical considerations.

One consequence of the fact that monoclonal antibody production is labour intensive is that very few Mabs are commercially viable and, although increasing numbers are being marketed, they are very expensive. Many useful antigen specificities are not available commercially and, in any case, research laboratories generally find it cheaper to produce their own Mabs even when a particular specificity could be purchased 'off the shelf'. This raises an added complication: different laboratories may be identifying the *same* antigen with their locally produced Mabs, but there is no way of knowing this unless samples are traded and compared. Standardisation workshops are beginning to overcome this problem, and hybridoma 'banks' send deep-frozen hybridomas of known antigen specificity to laboratories around the world.

Another technical problem that remains to be solved is that although a great many mouse or rat Mabs with interesting or useful antigen specificities have been produced, it has proved much more difficult to produce *human* Mabs.

☐ Can you suggest why it is difficult to produce human Mabs?

■ There are two main problems. First, it is not usually acceptable to immunise human beings with antigens for commercial or research purposes, especially when repeated injections are necessary to produce high enough concentrations of activated B cells with the right specificity. Second, it is not acceptable to remove a person's spleen to obtain these cells, so they have to be isolated from samples of peripheral blood, which contains relatively few circulating plasma cells (as you will recall from Chapter 3).

The relative lack of human monoclonal antibodies has certain consequences for medical treatment and research, as you will see later in this Chapter. Nonetheless, the technique of using hybridomas to synthesise monoclonal antibodies has revolutionised methods for identifying and quantifying antigens, and resulted in a Nobel prize being awarded to Milstein and Köhler in 1984.

7.2   Antigen purification by immunoaffinity chromatography

We will not dwell on immunoaffinity chromatography, although it is an important method for purifying antigens, because you have already been introduced to the principle of it in reverse—when we discussed the purification of polyclonal antisera by adsorbing the wanted antibodies with the immunising antigen. When the *antigen* is the required product, the chromatography column contains agarose beads to which specific antibodies have been coupled by covalent bonds linking the Fc region of the antibody molecule to the solid support. The antigen of interest is 'captured' when a mixture containing it passes down the column. Both polyclonal and monoclonal antibody preparations are used in immunoaffinity chromatography, but Mabs have certain advantages.

☐ Can you suggest what they are?

■ Mabs have two main advantages. First, polyclonal antisera contain many different antibody specificities and are rarely free from contaminating antibodies, all of which become bound to the column. Even if the contaminants do not have binding sites for the antigen of interest, they dilute the antibodies that have the correct specificities (i.e. there are fewer 'traps' per column). In contrast, *all* the antibodies in a monoclonal preparation bind to the antigen of interest. Second, polyclonal antisera bind the antigen very tightly to the column because they bind to several different epitopes (i.e. they have high *avidity*); this makes it more difficult to release the antigen. In contrast, Mabs bind to a single epitope and so the affinity is generally lower and the antigen is more easily recovered. (However, some Mabs have such high affinity for their antigen that the antigen cannot easily be removed without denaturing it.)

Immunoaffinity chromatography is now widely used in research and, increasingly, in industrial and pharmaceutical chemistry to extract a particular antigen from a complex mixture, especially where the contaminating antigens are chemically similar to the antigen of interest. It is possible, using this method, to purify antigens in relatively large quantities compared with the amounts, in the region of a few micrograms, that most other methods yield. However, hospital pathology and biological research laboratories often require a method of separating antigens solely in order to identify and quantify them; they don't need to recover them in a pure form. It is to these methods that we now turn.

7.3 Precipitation of soluble antigens

A number of methods have been developed for detecting, identifying and quantifying soluble antigens by precipitating them out of solution as immune complexes. They use polyclonal antisera or Mabs combined in mixtures for the reasons discussed earlier. Precipitation methods are relatively cheap and easy to perform because there is a visible end-point and the equipment is simple. The methods can be made quantitative because the precipitate forms only when the concentration of antigen and the concentration of antibody are within certain limits. This is known as the **precipitin reaction**.

When a soluble *multivalent* antigen is mixed with a preparation of *divalent* antibodies, the concentration of each solution affects the extent of precipitate formation. If *antigen* is present in excess, then only a few of the available epitopes will be bound to antibodies, and relatively few molecules of antigen will be cross-linked to each other (Figure 7.2a). Conversely, if *antibodies* are present in excess, then most antibody molecules will have neither or only one of their binding sites filled by epitopes, and again rather few cross-links between antigen molecules can be formed (Figure 7.2c). Thus, precipitation of immune complexes only takes place when there is a rough *equivalence* between the number of available *epitopes* in the antigen solution and the number of available *binding sites* in the antibody solution (Figure 7.2b). This occurs at the so-called **equivalence point**, where immune complexes form extensively cross-linked *lattices* that are large enough to precipitate out of solution.

If the precipitin reaction occurs in an aqueous solution, the amount of immune complex present can be estimated by using a spectrophotometer to measure the extent to which light is scattered by the complexes in the solution. Other methods are based on precipitin reactions taking place in semi-solid gels.

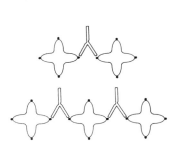

(a) antigen excess

(b) equivalence

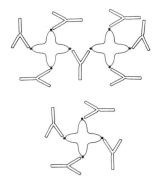

(c) antibody excess

FIGURE 7.2 Immune complexes formed between divalent antibodies with binding sites for (in this hypothetical case) an antigen with four identical epitopes. (a) The number of epitopes greatly exceeds the number of binding sites (i.e. antigen is in excess). (b) There is roughly the same number of epitopes as binding sites. (c) The number of binding sites greatly exceeds the number of epitopes (i.e. antibody is in excess). Notice that the immune complexes are small in (a) and (c) but that an extensive lattice of cross-linked antigen and antibody molecules can form at the equivalence point shown in (b).

7.3.1 Immunodiffusion methods

The basic principle of all **immunodiffusion** methods for detecting soluble antigens is that the antigen and the antibody solution diffuse towards each other through a thin layer of semi-solid gel, usually on a glass plate or shallow dish. After they meet, an appropriate concentration of each is reached (the equivalence point) and a visible precipitate forms. Visibility of the precipitin lines is sometimes improved by staining the gel with a protein-reactive dye, which binds to the immune complexes, and placing the plate over a light-box.

There are a number of variations on this basic theme. For example, in the *Ouchterlony diffusion* method, several different antigens (or antibody preparations) are applied to wells in the gel in different locations to identify which combinations interact. Only those antibodies and antigens with complementary binding sites will form a precipitate as they diffuse together.

In the **radial immunodiffusion** assay (or RID), either the antigen or the antibody solution is mixed with the molten gel so that the molecules are evenly dispersed through the gel when it is applied to the plate. Then one or more wells are cut in the gel and a solution of the other partner in the precipitin reaction is added. After a time, a radial precipitin ring forms around each well. Figure 7.3 shows a typical RID plate in which the antibodies are dispersed in the gel and serial dilutions of antigen have been added to wells cut in the plate.

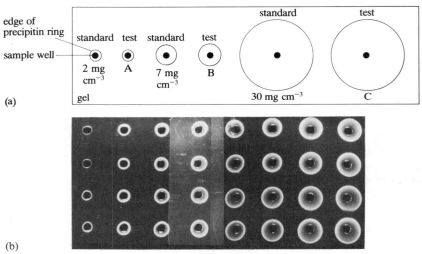

FIGURE 7.3 (a) Diagram of a radial immunodiffusion gel at the end-point of an assay to quantify IgG (the antigen) in the serum of patients A, B and C. Patients' serum is added to the test wells, the standard wells contain known concentrations of IgG for comparison, and the gel contains antibodies that bind to human IgG, raised in another species. The normal level of IgG in human serum is about 7 mg cm^{-3}, as in the sample taken from patient B. Patients A and C have, respectively, much lower or much higher IgG levels than normal. (b) Photograph of a radial immunodiffusion gel at the end-point of an assay. The gel contains a rabbit antiserum with binding sites for a polysaccharide (S3) derived from *Pneumococcus* bacteria. Samples of purified S3 are added to wells cut in the gel in increasing concentrations from top left to bottom right of the plate. After an appropriate incubation period, the plate is placed over a light box and the diameter of the precipitin rings is measured. A standard curve of antigen concentration plotted against ring diameter squared allows the quantification of bacterial antigen in test samples.

☐ Why doesn't the soluble antigen precipitate as soon as it meets the antibodies in the gel?

■ The antigen does not precipitate immediately because at first its concentration greatly exceeds the antibody concentration, but as it diffuses further from the well, the antigen concentration falls until the equivalence point is reached, and a ring of precipitate forms around the well.

RID assays are quantitative because the area within the radial precipitin ring is proportional to the concentration of antigen in the well. The concentration of a test sample can be estimated by reference to standard (known) concentrations of the *same* antigen added to wells in the same plate (as in Figure 7.3). RID assays are still much used in hospital laboratories because the method is simple and cheap, even though far more sensitive methods now exist. RID is used to estimate the concentration of certain known antigens that may appear in the serum or urine of patients. Such antigens include serum immunoglobulins or proteins that are excreted by patients with certain kinds of tumour or kidney disease. However, only one antigen can be tested for at a time, the method is slow (especially if the antigens or antibodies have a high M_r because they have slow diffusion rates), and mixtures of antigens cannot be separated unless the antigens differ significantly in mass. If the separation of antigens in complex mixtures is required, the simplest method is to use gel electrophoresis.

7.3.2 Immunoelectrophoresis methods

Proteins with different net charges can be separated in a gel by electrophoresis. An electric current is applied to the gel and the proteins separate because they migrate at different rates towards the positive or negative pole (the rates also depend on the pH of the gel). This has been exploited in **immunoelectrophoresis**, a two-stage method in which a mixture of protein antigens is first separated by electrophoresis in a thin layer of agarose gel on a glass plate. In the second stage, a trough is cut in the plate and a solution of specific antibodies is added. These diffuse towards the separated antigens and form arcs of precipitated immune complexes at the equivalence points (Figure 7.4).

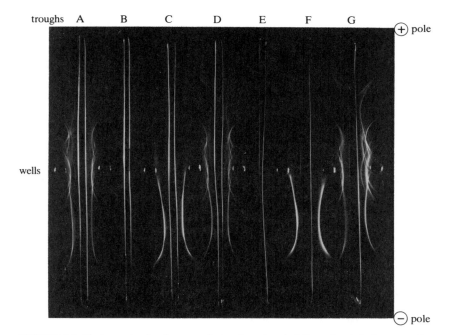

FIGURE 7.4 Photograph of an immunoelectrophoresis gel at the end-point of an assay for human serum proteins (the antigens), which were added to the circular wells before the current was applied. After electrophoretic separation, troughs A to G were cut in the gel and antisera were added. A, D and G contained a polyspecific antiserum to whole human serum proteins; C and F contained an antiserum that binds to human IgG heavy chains; B and E contained an antiserum that binds weakly to a β-globulin. Notice the symmetrical precipitin arcs on either side of each trough. The very long arc pointing towards the negative pole on either side of troughs C and F results from the wide range of charge (and hence electrophoretic mobility) in the IgG fraction of human serum due to variability in the structures of the antigen binding sites. The arcs have been made more visible by placing the gel on a light box.

Alternatively, the antibodies are mixed with the gel beforehand, and the pH is chosen so that the antibodies have no net charge and thus remain stationary when the current is applied. At this pH the antigens are negatively charged. When the antigens are added to wells cut in the gel at the negative pole of the plate, they migrate towards the anode into the antibody-containing gel (Figure 7.5). Because of the enforced direction of migration, the precipitin lines that form at the equivalence points are rocket shaped, giving this method its name—**rocket immunoelectrophoresis**. Since antibody concentration is uniform throughout the gel, the area under the rocket-shaped precipitin line is proportional to antigen concentration. Just as with immunodiffusion, these methods are most useful for well characterised antigens for which standard preparations of antisera of known concentration are available. They are faster than passive diffusion methods but they cannot separate antigens that have very similar net charges. An alternative method of separating proteins on the basis of their *mass* rather than their charge, and which also uses electrophoresis as its first step, is discussed in Section 7.5.3.

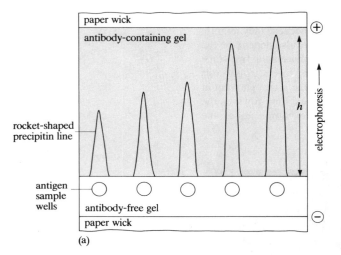
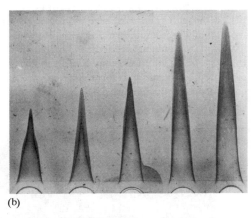

FIGURE 7.5 (a) Diagram of a rocket electrophoresis gel at the end-point of an assay. At the start of the assay, the wells contain known concentrations of an antigen and the gel contains specific antibodies that bind the antigen. A standard curve can be constructed by plotting the height of each rocket against the antigen concentration. The curve can then be used to estimate the concentration of test samples of the antigen. (b) Photograph of a rocket electrophoresis gel in which the precipitin lines have been stained with a protein-binding dye. In this example, the antigen is α-foetoprotein in the amniotic fluid of a 16 week human foetus. The four wells to the left of the gel contained increasing concentrations of antigen from the same sample and the well on the far right contained a normal standard sample of the antigen for comparison. The gel was mixed with a purified polyclonal antiserum that binds to α-foetoprotein. Raised levels of α-foetoprotein may indicate that the foetus is affected by spina bifida.

7.4 Agglutination of cell-bound antigens

Antigens on the surface of cells can be detected by polyclonal antisera (or mixtures of Mabs), which agglutinate the cells into visible clumps. This method is used to some extent to detect naturally occurring cell-surface antigens, but it is far more commonly used for cells that have been artificially coated with either an antigen or an antibody preparation, which has been covalently coupled to the cell membrane. Red blood cells are most frequently used in **agglutination tests** because their colour makes them visible and so the difference between a positive and a negative result is immediately apparent, as Figure 7.6 shows.

In Figure 7.6, the red cells have been coated with antigen, and *haem*agglutination indicates the presence of specific antibodies in the antiserum. The red cell agglutination method can be reversed so that antibodies in a standard preparation are coupled to the red cells by their Fc regions, and the cells are then agglutinated in the presence of a specific antigen. The method can be made quantitative by comparing the haemagglutination produced by serial dilutions of the test sample of antigen or antibody with that produced by a standard sample.

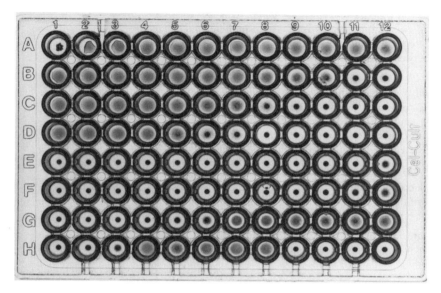

FIGURE 7.6 Haemagglutination microtitration plate at the end-point of an assay. Each well contains a standard suspension of sheep red blood cells coated with human serum albumin (HSA, the antigen). Rows A to D contain anti-HSA antiserum in increasing dilutions across the plate from left to right and down the rows from top to bottom (thus, the most concentrated solution of antiserum is in well A1 and the most dilute is in well D8). Wells D9 to D12 are controls without added antiserum. Wells in which the antibody concentration is high enough to agglutinate the red cells into a lattice show a diffuse uniform 'carpet' of cells across the concave bottom of the well; in the absence of sufficient antibody-binding, the red cells remain as single particles and slide down the sloping base of the well to form a tight pellet. Rows E to H contain a standard solution of anti-HSA antibodies and increasing dilutions of HSA (from left to right and from top to bottom); at high concentrations, the HSA inhibits the agglutination of the antigen-coated red cells by the antibodies. Wells H7 and H8 are controls without added free HSA, and H9 to H12 are controls without added antiserum.

7.5 Immunolabelling methods

In precipitation and agglutination methods there is a visible outcome of the antibody–antigen interaction, but these methods are often slow to produce a result and they are sometimes insufficiently sensitive or quantitative. The use of mono-clonal antibodies greatly increases the sensitivity and specificity of methods for detecting or assaying antigens, but Mabs are generally poor at forming precipitates or agglutinates. A number of methods have been developed to overcome this problem. They all employ a readily detectable label that is covalently linked *directly* to appropriate antibodies or antigens (Figure 7.7a and b), or to a second molecule that binds to the Fc region of the antibodies in the immune complex and labels the complex *indirectly* (Figure 7.7c, d and e). *Direct* **immunolabelling** is used in competitive inhibition assays, in which a known concentration of the labelled reagent competes with an unlabelled test sample of the *same* reagent for binding sites on the other partner in the immune complex. *Indirect* immunolabelling usually employs either anti-immunoglobulin antibodies (raised by injecting the antibodies of one species into another species, where they are recognised as foreign antigens) or *protein A* extracted from the cell wall of *Staphylococcus aureus*, which has a binding site for the Fc region of most subclasses of IgG. These indirect labelling methods are sometimes referred to as *sandwich* methods, because the molecules of interest are sandwiched between the solid matrix and the labelling agent.

Notice that in all these methods, one of the partners in the immune complex is always *fixed* to a solid support. It may, for example, be adsorbed on to the walls of small wells in a moulded plastic plate (called a *microtitration plate*; shown in Figure 7.6). In addition, the label is always linked to the *soluble* partner or to the second molecule. The assay depends on detecting and quantifying the label bound to the immune complexes.

☐ What is the *relationship* between the concentration of the test reagent and the amount of bound label at the end of the assay, in each of the combinations shown in Figure 7.7?

■ In (a) and (b) the amount of bound label is *inversely* proportional to the concentration of test sample, whereas in (c), (d) and (e) it is *directly* proportional.

The most common types of label used in quantitative assays are *radioactive* molecules and *enzymes*. The basic principle of the assay is the same whatever the nature of the label, so we will describe the assays that use radioactive labels in some detail and then briefly review the assays that use enzyme labels.

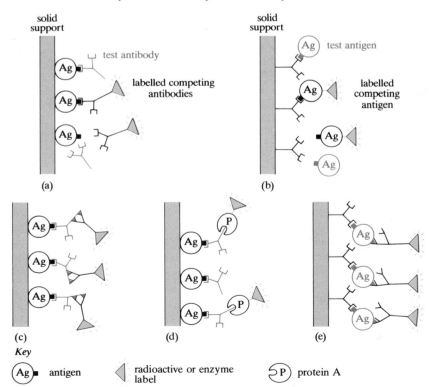

FIGURE 7.7 Immunolabelling methods for assaying antigens or antibodies. (a) and (b) are *direct* labelling methods, where the concentration of the test sample (red) of an antibody (a) or an antigen (b) is determined by competitive inhibition from a known concentration of the same reagent linked to a readily detectable label. (c), (d) and (e) are *indirect* labelling methods, where the test reagent (red) is 'sandwiched' between the solid-phase reagent and the labelling reagent. In (c) the labelling reagent is a second antibody, which binds to the Fc region of the test antibody; in (d) it is labelled protein A, which also binds to the Fc region of the test antibody; in (e) it is a second antibody with binding sites for a second epitope on the test antigen.

7.5.1. Radioimmunoassays

In the standard solid-phase **radioimmunoassay** (RIA), unlabelled antibodies with binding sites for the antigen of interest are coupled to a solid support—generally a plastic tube—and serial dilutions of the test sample of antigen (also unlabelled) are added as in Figure 7.8a. The concentration of the antigen in the test sample is estimated by *competitive inhibition* with a standard sample of radiolabelled antigen molecules added in a known concentration. The higher the concentration of the test antigen, the lower the final concentration of labelled standard antigens that will be bound to the antibodies, and the lower the radioactivity of the solid support at the end of the assay.

A calibration curve, such as the one shown in Figure 7.8b, is drawn from the results. The percentage of bound label is plotted against known concentrations of

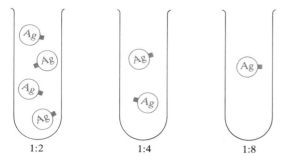

1:2   1:4   1:8

Step I: take known dilutions of unlabelled antigen

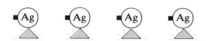

Step II: add standard concentration of radioactively-labelled antigens to each tube

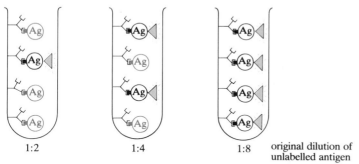

1:2   1:4   1:8   original dilution of unlabelled antigen

Step III: add mixture of unlabelled and labelled antigens to solid-phase antibodies with specific binding sites for the antigen; then wash out unbound antigens

Step IV: measure bound radioactivity for each antigen dilution

(a)

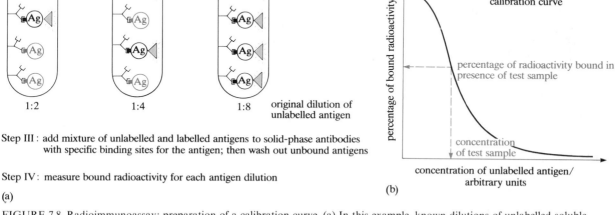

(b)

FIGURE 7.8 Radioimmunoassay: preparation of a calibration curve. (a) In this example, known dilutions of unlabelled soluble antigen are mixed with a standard concentration of the *same* antigen linked to a radioactive label. A competitive inhibition assay is set up in which labelled and unlabelled antigen molecules compete for binding sites on solid-phase antibodies. (The assay can be performed the other way round, i.e. with labelled and unlabelled soluble antibodies competing for epitopes on solid-phase antigens.) When unbound antigen molecules are washed away, the bound radioactivity is *inversely* proportional to the concentration of the soluble reagent. (b) A calibration curve is drawn from the results of a standard assay, such as the one shown in (a). The curve can be used to determine the concentration of a *test* sample of the unlabelled antigen. This is done by measuring the percentage of radioactivity that remains bound to the solid-phase antibody in the presence of the test sample, and reading the corresponding unlabelled antigen concentration from the curve.

the antigen in question. This can be used to determine the concentration of test samples of the antigen. It is vital for the accuracy of the assay that labelled and unlabelled antigens have exactly the same affinity for the antibodies, so the process by which the isotope is attached to the antigen must not affect the conformation of the epitope. Common radiolabelling agents are radioactive H, C or I atoms, which all cause comparatively small structural changes to the antigen. The basic RIA method is extremely sensitive and can assay protein antigens down to concentrations of about 10^{-12} g ml^{-1}. It has proved to be an invaluable method for detecting some cancer-associated proteins and hepatitis antigens in patient's serum, for monitoring the levels of certain drugs, and for detecting perturbations of normal hormone levels.

The method can be turned around to estimate the concentration of *antibodies* with binding sites for a particular antigen. In this case, the antigen is fixed to the solid support and is then reacted with unlabelled antibodies (from a patient's serum for example), in competition with labelled antibodies, as shown in Figure 7.7a. Alternatively, the amount of bound antibody can be estimated *indirectly* by attaching either radioactively-labelled anti-immunoglobulin antibodies from another species that bind to human Fc regions (as in Figure 7.7c), or radioactively-labelled protein A (Figure 7.7d).

Two modifications of the RIA method for detecting antibodies have major significance for **allergy** sufferers, who synthesise large amounts of IgE with binding sites for certain common, non-infectious environmental proteins, such as pollens. Proteins that elicit an allergic response in sensitised individuals are known as **allergens**. Desensitisation treatment requires the identification of the allergen to which the patient's IgE binds (and hence the allergen that triggers mast cell degranulation; see Section 2.4). In the **radioallergosorbent test (RAST)**, suspected allergens are covalently linked to cellulose discs, which are reacted with the patient's serum. Allergens that bind IgE from the patient's serum can be identified by indirect radiolabelling, using radioactively labelled anti-human-IgE antibodies (usually raised in rabbits). Much higher concentrations of the suspected allergens can be coupled to a paper disk that can be adsorbed on to the surface of plastic plates, and this is essential for detecting the very low concentrations of serum IgE (see Table 4.1). Note that the allergic reaction is not mediated by *serum* IgE but by IgE attached to mast cells (a subject to which we will return in Chapter 10).

The **radioimmunosorbent test (RIST)** measures the total concentration of IgE in the patient's serum, regardless of its antigen specificity. A plastic tube is first coated with rabbit anti-human-IgE antibodies, which are covalently linked to the plastic via their Fc regions. When patient's serum is added, the patient's IgE molecules are bound by the rabbit antibodies. If radioactively-labelled human IgE molecules are also added in known concentrations, then a competitive inhibition assay (akin to the situation shown in Figure 7.8) is set up. The *more* IgE that is present in the patient's serum, the *less* labelled, standard IgE will be bound to the rabbit antibodies and trapped on the plastic. Thus, a patient's IgE concentration is inversely proportional to bound radioactivity at the end of the assay.

7.5.2   Enzyme-linked assays

The methods just discussed for assaying antigens and antibodies using radioactive labels have been very successfully adapted by substituting particular *enzymes* for the isotope. Although the labelling agent is now a whole protein, the principle of the method is very similar. The *unlabelled* partner in the antigen–antibody interaction is attached to a solid matrix, and the assay can be performed either way round (i.e. with solid-phase antibodies to detect the presence of a certain antigen, or vice versa). The enzyme label is linked either to the soluble partner in the interaction, or to a second antibody or protein A. Commonly used enzymes include β-galactosidase, alkaline phosphatase and horse-radish peroxidase. The concentration of enzyme bound to the immune complex is estimated by the addition of its substrate and, sometimes, an indicator that changes colour when the substrate is acted on by the enzyme. Enzyme–substrate–indicator combinations that give a readily measurable coloured product are chosen.

An important and widely used assay method of this type is known as the **enzyme-linked immunosorbent assay**, or **ELISA** for short. The enzyme can be linked either to the antigen molecules or to the antibodies, but in either case the solid-phase reactant is *unlabelled*. ELISA can be made quantitative by setting it up as a competitive inhibition assay in which free antigen (or antibody) competes with enzyme-linked antigen (or antibody) for binding sites on the solid-phase reactant (Figure 7.9a and b), or by using the *test* sample in the solid-phase (Figure 7.9c). The principle is the same as that already discussed for assays using radioactively-labelled antigens or antibodies. The advantages of ELISA are that it is very sensitive (down to about 10^{-9} g ml^{-1}), the technique is simple, the end-point is reached quickly, enzymes are cheaper and more stable than isotopes, and there are none of the hazards of handling isotopes that accompany radioimmunoassays. However, the very high sensitivity of radioimmunoassays makes them the method of choice where sensitivity is the overriding consideration.

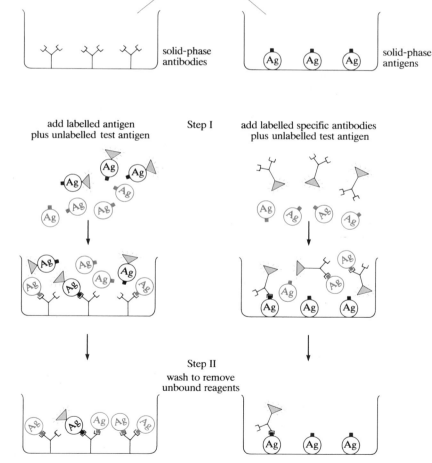

FIGURE 7.9 Competitive ELISA (enzyme-linked immunosorbent assay) for estimating the concentration of an unlabelled test sample of soluble antigen: (a) using enzyme-labelled antigen in competition with the test antigen for binding sites on solid-phase antibodies, and (b) using solid-phase antigen which competes with the test antigen for binding sites on soluble, enzyme-labelled antibodies. In both (a) and (b) the concentration of bound enzyme (and hence the amount of substrate converted to coloured product) is *inversely* proportional to the concentration of antigen in the test sample. (*Figure 7.9c is overleaf.*)

103

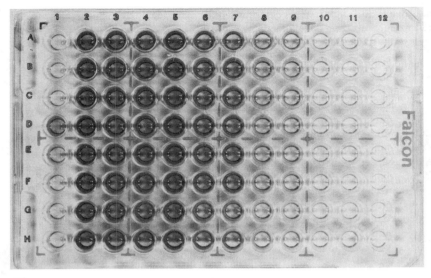

(c)

FIGURE 7.9(c) Photograph of a *non*-competitive ELISA microtitration plate at the end-point of an assay. The wells are first coated with test antigen (in this case a neuropeptide extracted from homogenised brain). The antigen is in serial dilutions down the plate, with the most concentrated solution in the top row and the most dilute in the bottom row. Then serial dilutions of an enzyme-linked antiserum that binds to the neuropeptide are added to the wells, with the most concentrated solution to the left of the plate and the most dilute to the right. When an appropriate substrate is added, a coloured product forms. In a non-competitive assay such as this, the amount of coloured product is *directly proportional* to the amount of immune complex formed in the well and hence to the amount of test antigen bound to the plastic.

7.5.3 Immunoblotting

Radioactive or enzyme-labelled antibodies are now frequently used to identify antigens that have first been separated by gel electrophoresis and then transferred to nitrocellulose paper. This method is far more sensitive than identification by precipitation of immune complexes in the gel (described earlier), and it allows monoclonal antibodies to be used, which are poor precipitators of antigen. **Immunoblotting** was developed to overcome the problem of co-migrating protein antigens (those with similar net charges). These proteins can be separated by gel electrophoresis, but only under conditions that cause denaturation. In this method, the electrophoresis is performed in a polyacrylamide gel containing sodium dodecyl sulphate (SDS), which imparts a strong and uniform negative charge to the proteins. This causes them to separate according to their *mass* when the current is applied and enables a much higher degree of separation to be achieved.

☐ What effect do you think the strong negative charge will have on the ability of specific antibodies to bind to the separated antigens in the gel?

■ Immune complexes will not be able to form because the normal patterns of charge are disrupted and this interferes with the non-covalent bonding between the epitope and the antigen binding sites of the antibody molecules.

Thus, the separated antigens are transferred on to wet, buffered nitrocellulose paper where their native conformation is restored. The transfer is carried out either by *pressure blotting*, that is, passive transfer of the antigen 'blots' on to paper that is applied with pressure to the gel (just like using blotting paper on wet ink) or, more commonly, by applying a second electric current across the gel at right angles to the first current (Figure 7.10a) so that the antigen 'blots' migrate on to the paper. This double electrophoresis method is known as *electroblotting*, and was first

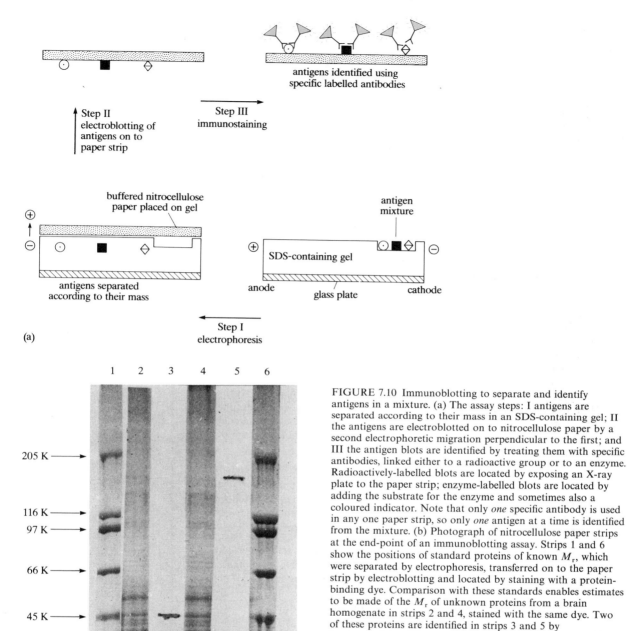

FIGURE 7.10 Immunoblotting to separate and identify antigens in a mixture. (a) The assay steps: I antigens are separated according to their mass in an SDS-containing gel; II the antigens are electroblotted on to nitrocellulose paper by a second electrophoretic migration perpendicular to the first; and III the antigen blots are identified by treating them with specific antibodies, linked either to a radioactive group or to an enzyme. Radioactively-labelled blots are located by exposing an X-ray plate to the paper strip; enzyme-labelled blots are located by adding the substrate for the enzyme and sometimes also a coloured indicator. Note that only *one* specific antibody is used in any one paper strip, so only *one* antigen at a time is identified from the mixture. (b) Photograph of nitrocellulose paper strips at the end-point of an immunoblotting assay. Strips 1 and 6 show the positions of standard proteins of known M_r, which were separated by electrophoresis, transferred on to the paper strip by electroblotting and located by staining with a protein-binding dye. Comparison with these standards enables estimates to be made of the M_r of unknown proteins from a brain homogenate in strips 2 and 4, stained with the same dye. Two of these proteins are identified in strips 3 and 5 by immunostaining. The paper was treated with an enzyme-linked monoclonal antibody to known brain proteins, and the blots were then visualised by adding the appropriate substrate. The 45 000 M_r protein in strip 3 is actin, a constituent of most cells, and the 170 000 M_r protein in strip 5 is a brain-specific protein.

developed by Ed Southern in Edinburgh for detecting DNA fragments separated by electrophoresis (it is called *Southern blotting* after its inventor). Since then, the method has been extended to the separation of RNA fragments (called *Northern* blotting) and proteins (*Western* blotting). (*Eastern* blotting has not yet been invented!) Immunoblotting is another name for Western blotting. Once the antigen blots have been transferred to the paper, they are identified and visualised by treating them with enzyme-linked antibodies and a suitable substrate (Figure 7.10b), or with radioactively-labelled antibodies and subsequent exposure of the paper strip to an X-ray plate.

7.5.4 Immunohistochemistry

Immunohistochemistry uses labelled antibodies to locate antigens or patient's antibodies in sections of tissue or on the surface of cells. Enzyme-labelled antibodies can be detected by the formation of a coloured product in the tissue section (for example, see Plate 8.1a). Radioactively-labelled antibodies are located by exposing an X-ray plate to the radioactive emissions from a section of treated tissue. But perhaps the most common method used in immunohistochemistry is **immunofluorescence**. It uses antibodies linked to fluorescent molecules either directly or via an intermediary, e.g. fluorescently-labelled second antibody or protein A. The patterns of fluorescence are visible when the treated tissue or cells are viewed under a fluorescence microscope (for example, see Plate 8.1b).

Antibodies linked to enzymes or to radioactive or fluorescent molecules have added important new staining techniques to the histochemist's repertoire, and have proved to be especially useful in characterising autoantibodies and their target antigens in autoimmune diseases.

7.5.5 Leukocyte assays using labelled antibodies

Labelled monoclonal antibodies have also been invaluable in identifying, separating and quantifying different types of leukocyte by binding to characteristic cell-surface marker molecules such as sIg, CD4 and CD8, or to the T cell receptor for antigen. They are also very useful in identifying cell function by binding to proteins secreted by a certain cell type. The surface molecules on leukocytes are immunogenic if presented correctly to a suitable responder animal, and highly specific Mabs with binding sites for leukocyte receptor molecules now exist. (In fact, in many cases the existence of these receptor molecules was inferred from the fact that specific Mabs were induced when leukocyte cell membranes were used as immunogens. When detected by Mabs these molecules are often referred to as leukocyte *antigens*, but you should be clear that they are, in fact, receptor molecules on the cells of the host animal.)

Labelled Mabs that bind to leukocyte receptors have enabled the *in vitro* study of immune-cell function to make rapid progress by offering ways to enrich leukocyte suspensions with, or deplete them of, cells of a particular type. The leukocyte population can also be characterised in patients with certain immune deficiency diseases or white cell cancers such as the leukaemias and lymphomas.

The most sensitive of the methods currently available is **flow cytofluorography**, which measures the fluorescence emitted by leukocytes that have been treated with, and have bound to, fluorescently-labelled Mabs. The cells are suspended in a buffered solution and pumped through a cytofluorograph machine under pressure. They emerge in a fine stream that passes through the path of a laser beam. The laser light energises the fluorescent molecules, which emit energy, and a sensor picks up each pulse and counts the number of cells with fluorescent Mabs attached. The machine also measures the extent to which the laser light is scattered and calculates the size of the cells from these data. Two types of Mabs can be used on the same leukocyte suspension, each with binding sites for a different surface receptor and each with a different fluorescent molecule attached. This is known as two-colour cytofluorography. The machine distinguishes between the different wavelengths emitted by the two fluorescent labels.

☐ How would you compare the number of helper T cells with the number of non-helper T cells using two-colour cytofluorography?

■ You would need two different Mabs, one with binding sites for CD4 (the marker for helper T cells) and one that binds to CD8 (the marker for cytotoxic cells and at least some of the suppressor-cell subset). Each of the Mabs would be linked to a different fluorescent label, and the cytofluorograph machine would count the number of cells in the population that carried either of these receptors in its surface membrane. (In fact, this method is used to track the decline in helper:suppressor ratio that characterises the onset of illness in patients infected with HIV, the human immunodeficiency virus.)

A variant of the cytofluorograph is the **fluorescence activated cell sorter** (or FACS machine), which has the additional property of physically *separating* cells bound to fluorescent Mabs from those that do not fluoresce and which, therefore, do not carry the surface antigen of interest. The stream emerging from the nozzle of the machine passes between electrically charged plates and the fluorescent cells are deflected by the electric field. Fluorescent and non-fluorescent cells are deflected to different degrees, so the stream is split and different subsets of leukocytes can be collected in enriched fractions. Cytofluorography techniques have enabled rapid progress to be made in investigating the functions of different subsets of lympho- cytes and their interactions in the immune response.

7.6   Rosettes and plaques

In the previous Section we looked at a method for identifying leukocytes of a particular subset by using labelled antibodies. The two methods described briefly here are alternative ways of distinguishing between T cells and B cells without using added antibodies. Both methods allow a reasonable estimate to be made of the number of cells.

The **T cell rosette assay** depends on the fact that human T cells have a peptide in their surface membrane that binds to a ligand on the surface of sheep red blood cells. (Although not relevant to the assay, you will doubtless be curious about this receptor! The T cell peptide has been given the designation CD2 and its function is to act as a receptor for a ligand that occurs on most other cells in the body, enabling the two cells to adhere to each other while other receptor–ligand interactions take place. The fact that this ligand also occurs on sheep red blood cells is either coincidental or, perhaps, a consequence of a common ancestral gene.) When human leukocytes are mixed with sheep red blood cells, the T cells bind to the red cells forming a rosette of lymphocytes around a central red cell. Rosettes can be counted under the light microscope and, because of their high density, can be removed from the leukocyte suspension by layering the cells on to a Ficoll density-gradient. Ficoll is a polymer that can be diluted with buffer to give solutions of known density. A density gradient can be built up by pouring layers of Ficoll of *decreasing* density into a tube. The cell suspension is poured on to the top of the gradient and the tube is centrifuged. The cells sink through the Ficoll until they reach a layer with a density that corresponds to their own.

☐   Where will the T cell rosettes be found in such a gradient?

■   At the bottom, because agglutinated cells have a much higher density than single cells.

This method can be used to separate T cells from a leukocyte suspension. Alternatively, the red cells can be covalently linked to Mabs that bind to specific leukocyte receptors (e.g. CD4 or CD8), so that artificially-induced rosettes form. This is quite a popular method for depleting a leukocyte population of a particular subset of white cells; the receptor-positive cells can be removed in rosettes by centrifugation, leaving the population of receptor-negative cells behind.

Red cells are also the target in a simple assay for B cells—the **B cell plaque-forming assay**. This assay identifies B cells that have a particular antigen specificity and so is unlike the T rosette methods described above, which identify T cells *regardless* of their antigen specificity. Activated B cells can be identified by their ability to produce antibodies that will lyse red cells in the presence of complement. The red cells are first coated with the antigen of interest and then mixed with the leukocyte suspension and complement. The concentration of red cells is carefully adjusted so that a monolayer of cells is formed when the suspension is placed between two glass plates. At first, the monolayer appears uniformly red, but after incubating it at an appropriate temperature for several hours 'holes', or *plaques*, appear in it as red cells in these locations are lysed. The plaques form around plasma cells that are secreting antibodies with binding sites for the antigen on the red cells; the antibodies activate the complement cascade and this results in red cell lysis.

There are many other methods for determining the function or estimating the numbers of particular leukocyte cell types. Some use antibodies to identify characteristic molecules on the cell surface or to detect proteins secreted by the cell. Others, the so-called *bioassays*, expose the cells *in vitro* to activating signals such as antigens, interleukins or mitogens, and then measure the extent of cell division that follows. We have no space to go into further details of these methods here (reference manuals are included in the Further Reading section at the end of this Book), but the selection in this Chapter should have given you a reasonable understanding of some of the most important uses of antibodies in detecting antigens in the laboratory. We finish the Chapter with a brief look at some of the current uses of antibodies, not in the laboratory but in human patients.

7.7   Diagnostic and therapeutic uses of antibodies *in vivo*

Protective antibodies are elicited by infection and immunisation, but in this Section we will focus on pre-formed antibodies that are injected into patients as diagnostic or therapeutic tools. The main target in all these studies has been cancer cells. The passive injection of antibodies for cancer therapy has proved to be disappointing so far. More promising have been techniques in which a radioactive molecule, toxin or cytotoxic drug is attached to the Fc region of antibodies that are directed against epitopes on malignant cells, and then injected into the patient where it 'homes in' on the affected tissue. The tissue may then be located by detecting the radioactivity; alternatively, the radioactive dose or drug may (in theory) be lethal to the malignant cells. This has given rise to the expectation that anti-cancer antibodies will prove to be 'magic bullets' that doctors can 'fire' at cancers without bystander damage to non-malignant tissue in their patients. However, there are still a number of serious problems to be overcome.

Monoclonal antibodies have proved to be more successful than polyclonal antisera in targetting drugs or isotopes on to cancer cells because of their greater epitope specificity, but progress has been hindered by the difficulty of producing human hybridomas (for the reasons discussed earlier in this Chapter). If mouse or rat Mabs are injected into a human patient, within a short time the patient will begin to secrete antibodies directed against epitopes in the rodent immunoglobulins, so their use is generally limited to single treatments and diagnostic applications. Figure 7.11 shows the use of a radioactively-labelled Mabs from a rat hybridoma to identify tumour deposits in the lungs of a human patient.

A solution to this problem may come from genetic engineering. It has already proved possible to splice the DNA sequences that code for the hypervariable loops of rat antibodies into the genome of human B cells. When these cells are fused into hybridomas, the antibodies that they secrete have the conformation of human immunoglobulins in all of their structure except for the antigen binding site, which is derived from the rat genome. This opens the door to custom-built monoclonal antibodies of the future. However, it does not solve the problem that suitable epitopes are difficult to find on cancer cells. Most of the epitopes on human cancer cells that are candidates for binding by monoclonal antibodies also occur on other cell types, so the danger of cross-reactivity with normal tissue is high. This presents an unacceptable risk if the anti-cancer Mabs are linked to a highly radioactive or cytotoxic molecule.

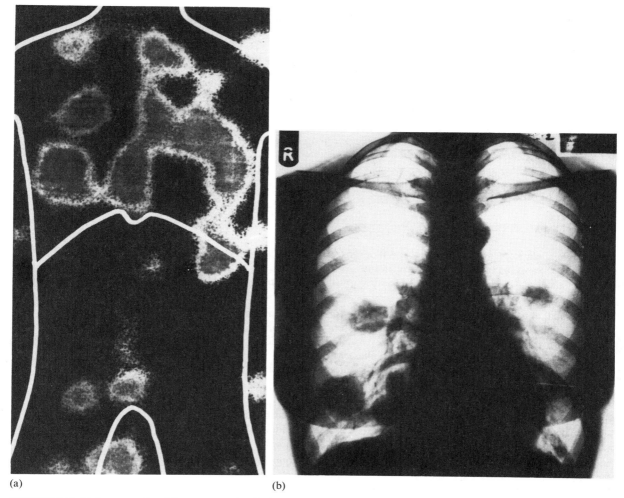

(a)   (b)

FIGURE 7.11 (a) Image produced by an external radiation camera showing the location (bright patches) of radioactively-labelled Mabs obtained from a rat hybridoma, which bind to colon cancer cells in a human patient. The original cancer in the large intestine was removed surgically several years previously; the distribution of isotope here indicates that cancer cells have spread to form new tumours, principally in the chest. (The image is produced in colour, not black and white as here, and is colour-coded to indicate which areas have bound most radioactive isotope. The camera also detects some radiation 'scattered' outside the patient's body, hence the superimposed outline.) (b) X-ray plate taken of the chest of the same patient confirming the presence of 'cannonball' deposits of cancer cells (dark patches) growing in the lungs.

Some success has been reported in the use of Mabs to overcome the hitherto serious problem of using donated bone marrow to reconstitute patients who have been given whole-body irradiation. Patients with leukaemias and some other cancers may sometimes be cured by irradiating them to destroy all their white cells (normal and malignant), and then reconstituting them with normal bone marrow. The irradiation process itself causes damage to normal tissues, but more serious problems can arise from even small mismatches between the MHC molecules on the cells of the patient and those on the cells of the bone marrow donor.

☐   Can you predict what may happen when a mismatched bone marrow graft is injected into an irradiated patient?

■   Some of the immunologically active white cells in the bone marrow graft will have receptors for epitopes in the MHC molecules of the patient's cells (remember from Chapter 4 that some of these molecules were originally known as transplantation antigens). As MHC molecules are found on virtually every cell in the body, the donated lymphocytes will generate a widespread immune response against the patient's cells.

This condition is known as **graft versus host disease** and unless it is controlled by immunosuppressive drugs, the patient may die from the effects of the graft response. One way around this is to remove a sample of the patient's *own* bone marrow before the irradiation, and then use it later for the graft. The bone marrow will be contaminated with cancer cells, but they may be removed by mixing the marrow with tiny magnetic beads that have been coated with cancer-specific Mabs. The bone marrow is then passed between strong electromagnets which trap the beads and the cancer cells that have become bound to them. The 'clean' bone marrow is then re-injected into the patient. The early results of trials of bone marrow grafting using this technique have been very encouraging.

Summary of Chapter 7

1   Polyclonal antisera and monoclonal antibodies (Mabs) are used widely in industrial processes, in biological research, in medical diagnosis and, to a lesser extent, in medical treatment, to identify, localise, purify or quantify particular antigens or antibodies.

2   Polyclonal antisera are generally preferred to Mabs if the assay method relies on the ability to precipitate soluble antigens out of solution in immune complexes, or to agglutinate cell-bound antigens; but polyclonal antisera generally require purification to remove contaminating antibodies. Mabs have the significant advantages of being pure preparations of antibodies with a known antigen specificity and affinity, of being a single immunoglobulin class, and of being available (at least in theory) in unlimited amounts.

3   Antibodies (and especially Mabs) are used in immunoaffinity chromatography to extract and purify antigens from complex mixtures of similar molecules.

4   A number of assays for antigens or antibodies in solution exploit the precipitin reaction, in which immune complexes precipitate at the equivalence point. Precipitation may follow passive diffusion in gels (immunodiffusion methods), or electrophoretic separation (immunoelectrophoresis methods).

5   Agglutination methods use the visible end-point of cells agglutinated by cross-linking antibodies. Red cells are commonly used in agglutination methods after coating them with antigens or antibodies.

6   In several types of assay, antigens or antibodies are detected and quantified by reacting them with labelled partners in immune complexes. The labels may be radioactive isotopes, fluorescent molecules or enzymes, and are linked to either partner in the complex, to a second antibody, or to protein A. These methods can be made quantitative using competitive inhibition between the test sample of antigen (or antibody) and a standard solution of its labelled equivalent.

7   Immunohistochemistry employs antibodies, second antibodies or protein A with radioactive, fluorescent or enzyme labels to localise particular antigens or autoantibodies in tissue sections and on cells.

8   Cells of different immunological types can be identified, counted or separated by flow cytofluorography using fluorescent Mabs directed against cell-surface receptors, or by T cell rosette or B cell plaque-forming assays.

9   Cancer-specific Mabs from rodent hybridomas and, increasingly, from human hybridomas can be used to diagnose and localise tumours via radioactive labels attached to the antibodies. There is potential for targeting therapeutically useful doses of radioactivity, drugs or toxins using these antibodies *in vivo*, or for 'cleaning up' a patient's bone marrow *in vitro* before returning it to the patient.

Now attempt SAQs 25–29, which relate to this Chapter.

CHAPTER 8
MATURATION OF THE ADAPTIVE RESPONSE

In this Chapter we return to the adaptive immune response as it occurs in higher vertebrates, and describe the developmental sequence of the immune system as it matures from the embryo to the adult. In particular, we focus on the acquisition of **immune competence**, i.e. the ability to mount an effective immune response in which all the humoral and cell-mediated elements that we described in the preceding Chapters collaborate to protect the organism from infection. We are not born with full immune competence and having acquired it we may not retain it throughout life. Moreover, as the immune system matures it also has to acquire and maintain *self-tolerance*, that is, the *inability* to mount a damaging immune response against normal cells and molecules in the body.

8.1 Immune competence in embryos and new-born mammals

If you look back at Figure 2.2, you will see that all leukocytes develop from multipotent stem cells in the bone marrow and liver of the mammalian embryo, and that they continue to develop in adult bone marrow throughout life. In the human foetus, this process starts as early as the sixth week of gestation. By the eighth or ninth week the precursors of B cells can be detected in foetal liver, and later all the immunological cell types can be found in the circulation.

Although all the cells responsible for innate and adaptive immunity can be detected in the human foetus, some foetal cells are less able than their counterparts in the new-born baby to mount an immune response (i.e. they show less immune competence). Other cell types take one or even two years of life to mature to the level of competence that is seen in adults. For example, phagocytic cells in the foetus are less efficient at engulfing bacteria or other antigen particles than those in the new-born baby. However, this may in part be due to the lack of opsonising molecules in the foetal circulation. The components of complement do not begin to appear in the serum until about the second or third month of gestation (C3b is a powerful opsonin) and they reach only 50 to 60 per cent of the adult concentration by the time of birth. Similarly, IgM (another potent opsonin) is not synthesised by foetal B cells until about the fifth month of gestation, but maternal IgG crosses the placenta and enters the foetal circulation. Figure 8.1 shows how little antibody production there is in the new-born baby. Despite the rapid onset of IgG synthesis after birth, the concentration in the circulation does not reach the adult level until about two years of age, and IgA takes even longer to reach adult values.

It has also been shown that the ability of new-born rats to synthesise antibodies with binding sites for certain antigens develops *sequentially* during the first month of life. At birth, rats can produce antibodies to antigens in the cell walls of *Brucella abortus*, the bacteria that cause brucellosis, but not to several other antigens that have been tested experimentally. For example, they cannot produce antibodies to sheep red blood cells if this antigen is injected before the rats are three *days* old, and they must be about two *weeks* old before they can produce antibodies to polysaccharides in the capsule of *Streptococcus pneumoniae*. This suggests that rearrangement of the immunoglobulin V genes from the germ-line DNA is still going on in the maturing B cells after birth.

Throughout life, B cells and T cells continue to develop from stem cells in the bone marrow, topping up the circulating pool of immunocompetent lymphocytes as mature cells die. *Naive* B cells (i.e. mature cells with sIg receptors that have not come into contact with antigen) live only a few days, whereas memory B cells and all T cells live for months or years. Thus, in a discussion of the maturation of the immune response it is important to distinguish between the age of the *cell* and the age of the *animal* in which it is found. The sequence of maturation of both B and T cells occurs in two phases: the first is antigen-independent and the second is antigen-driven.

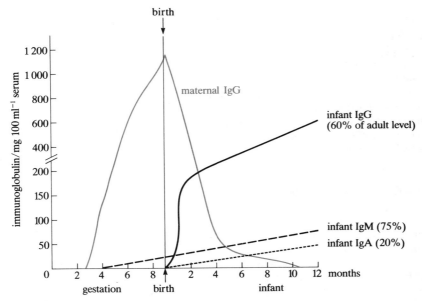

FIGURE 8.1 Serum immunoglobulin levels in the human foetus and in the first year after birth. Maternal IgG is passively acquired across the placenta before birth, and afterwards in colostrum and breastmilk. The figures in brackets are the percentage of adult levels of immunoglobulin found in infants at twelve months of age. (Notice that the vertical axis of this graph changes scale between 200 and 400 mg Ig per 100 ml serum.)

8.2 B cell maturation

Figure 8.2 summarises the appearance of immunoglobulins in the cytoplasm and then on the surface of B cell precursors as they mature independently of antigen. During the development of *pre*-B cells, recombination and rearrangement of the *variable* immunoglobulin genes for both the light and the heavy chains takes place (as described in Chapter 4). This generates millions of different B cell clones, each committed to produce antibodies with variable regions that recognise a particular epitope. Heavy chains of the IgM class can be detected in the cytoplasm of pre-B cells, and cells designated as *immature* B cells express surface IgM, together with class II MHC molecules and receptors for complement.

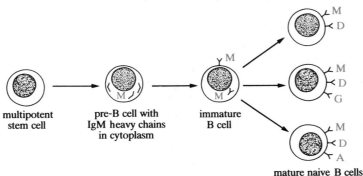

FIGURE 8.2 Maturation of B cells before contact with antigen. Letters in red denote the class of immunoglobulin detectable at each stage of development, either in the cytoplasm or on the surface membrane of the cell. (The very small numbers of mature B cells committed to IgE synthesis have been omitted.)

Note from Figure 8.2 that three types of *mature* B cell develop. All of these have surface IgM and IgD, but some also have IgG or IgA. It is possible for B cells to have surface immunoglobulin of more than one class. This is because all the heavy-chain constant-region genes remain intact in the B cell DNA (as described in Chapter 4), and mRNA transcripts of different heavy-chain genes can be spliced and translated into molecules of IgM, IgD, IgA or IgG. Even though the constant regions of surface immunoglobulins on a single mature B cell may differ, their variable regions are identical, and so they recognise the same epitope.

Clonal expansion and further development of the mature B cell takes place only after primary contact with antigen (Figure 8.3). Mature naive B cells that had only surface IgM and IgD are the main clones activated to differentiate into IgM-secreting plasma cells during the primary response. Plasma cells have very little surface immunoglobulin, whereas the memory cells that also differentiate at this time have a high concentration of sIg of the appropriate class but little or no sIgD. Many of the IgM memory cells formed during the primary response make the immunoglobulin class switch to produce IgG memory cells. Thus, if the same antigen is encountered a second time, the secondary antibody response is pre-dominantly of the IgG class. Most class switching is *irreversible* (that is, it involves deletion of heavy-chain genes from the B cell DNA), but there is evidence of switching back in at least some B cells. This suggests that some of the switching may be achieved at the level of the mRNA transcript.

☐ It is interesting to speculate about the function of class switching from IgM to IgG, i.e. from low-affinity, high-valency antibodies to high-affinity, low-valency antibodies. Can you suggest why such a switch might be advantageous?

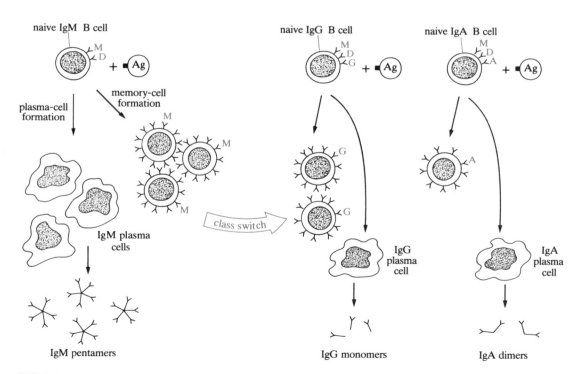

FIGURE 8.3 Antigen-dependent differentiation of B cells during the primary response to an antigen. Letters in red denote the class of surface-bound immunoglobulin (sIg); note that memory cells have abundant sIg but plasma cells have very little. The major class of secreted antibodies in serum during the primary response is IgM, but the concentration of IgG rises considerably during the secondary response because some IgM memory cells have switched class to IgG, increasing the pool of IgG memory cells. (A similar class switch to IgA and to IgE may also occur.)

■ Low-affinity receptors are likely to cross-react with a range of similar epitopes, and high valency presents a high concentration of binding sites that could aggregate antigens of various kinds. Therefore, IgM could function in a relatively generalised way as a recognition molecule for a range of similar antigens encountered for the first time. When a particular antigen *is* encountered, the class switch to IgG ensures that a more specific recognition molecule can be produced in response to it on any future exposure.

Finally, it is worth considering the immense scale of the expansion that takes place in a B cell clone after contact with antigen. It has been shown experimentally that, given the correct signals from helper T cells and optimum conditions *in vivo*, a single mature B cell from a mouse can multiply to produce 10^{10} daughter cells. Replication was exponential and the result implied that antigen-triggered clones of B cells will continue to replicate indefinitely unless regulated by inhibitory mechanisms (the subject of the next Chapter). Fortunately, such mechanisms exist and plasma cells die after the immune response to a particular antigen is complete, but the memory cells live on.

8.3   T cell maturation

T cells mature in the thymus gland in the mammalian embryo and young adults. But as mammals age, the need for the thymus as the site for T cell differentiation apparently declines, and it is possible to remove the gland from adults without loss of future T cell function. This seems to indicate that mature T cells survive a very long time, or even that they may be able to mature in the peripheral circulation later in life.

In the embryo of higher vertebrates, cells of the lymphoid type enter the thymus in waves at intervals of several days. After each wave has entered, no more cells can get into the thymus until the descendants of that wave of cells have either died in the thymus or emerged into the peripheral circulation. The cells that enter the thymus are apparently the same as the pre-B cells (or at least they have similar surface markers), so it is at least possible that prior to entering the thymus they could have been induced to differentiate into either B cells or T cells.

Once in the thymus, the developing T cells are referred to as **thymocytes**. They migrate through the thymus from the outer edge towards the centre of the gland, guided by the branched dendritic processes of thymic epithelial cells in the cortex and in the medulla, as shown in Figure 8.4. Thymocytes in the cortex are densely packed and rapidly dividing, but as they approach the junction between the cortex and the medulla large numbers of thymocytes die. The medulla contains fewer lymphocytes than the cortex but these have the characteristic surface markers of mature T cells.

During this journey through the thymus some cell surface markers are lost from the thymocytes and others are gained in a precise developmental sequence. For example, the peptide known as CD2 (which is involved in cell-to-cell adhesion interactions and is also the receptor for sheep red blood cells) first appears in the membrane of thymocytes that have newly arrived in the outer cortex. Later, CD4 and CD8 can be found *simultaneously* on thymocytes in the deeper cortex, but by the time they reach the medulla the mature T cells express *either* CD4 *or* CD8. Thus, the emergent T cells are already differentiated into subsets: CD4-positive cells display helper activity and CD8-positive cells display either cytotoxic or suppressor activity. (We return to the mechanisms that 'select' T cells for one subset or the other shortly.) However, **T cell subset differentiation** is not necessarily fixed for life. Several experiments have shown that helper T cells can, under certain conditions, act as suppressors of immune function. It may be that switching

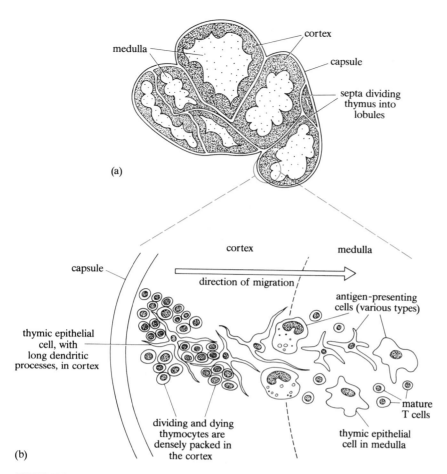

FIGURE 8.4 (a) Basic structure of the thymus gland. (b) Enlarged area of the gland showing zones of thymocyte maturation, proliferation and selection in the cortex and medulla. During their migration through the thymus, thymocytes that have binding sites for foreign antigen in association with self-MHC molecules are selected; thymocytes with binding sites for self-epitopes are probably deleted.

between activities contributes to the regulatory function of T cells—a subject to which we return in the next Chapter.

8.3.1 The acquisition of self-MHC restriction

The thymus is also the place where T cells acquire **self-MHC restriction**. The T cells that emerge from the thymus into the peripheral circulation can bind to antigens only when they are presented in association with the *same* MHC molecules that occur on the epithelial cells in the thymus in which they matured. The earliest experiment to demonstrate the importance of the thymus in self-MHC restriction was performed by Ralph Zinkernagel in 1978, and is summarised in Figure 8.5. He took two *congenic* strains of mouse (that is, strains that differed only in their *MHC* genes) and interbred them to produce hybrid offspring. The parents were from strains designated H-2^d and H-2^k, and the hybrid offspring expressed both sets of parental genes and were thus H-$2^{d/k}$. (H-2 is the name given to the *MHC* genes in mice, and ^{d} and ^{k} signify the specific *haplotypes* of the mice, that is, the different genes, in this case *MHC* genes, carried on a single chromosome.) Study the caption to Figure 8.5, which describes four steps in the experiment, involving the destruction of the thymus gland and the subsequent reconstitution of the hybrid mice with fresh bone marrow cells and a parental thymus graft.

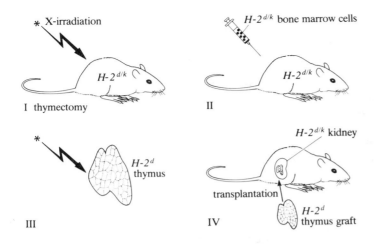

FIGURE 8.5 Protocol for an experiment showing that T cells acquire self-MHC restriction during their development in the thymus. I The thymus of an $H-2^{d/k}$ hybrid mouse is removed, and the mouse is then irradiated with X-rays. II The mouse is reconstituted with $H-2^{d/k}$ bone marrow cells. III An $H-2^d$ thymus is X-irradiated. IV The thymus is grafted into the $H-2^{d/k}$ mouse under the kidney capsule.

☐ Why did Zinkernagel irradiate the hybrid mice *and* the parental thymus grafts before performing the transplant (step IV)?

◼ The graft and the graft recipient already contained developing and mature T cells, which were destroyed by irradiation. The hybrid mouse could then be reconstituted with fresh bone marrow cells (that had not been through the thymus), and with a parental thymus gland that had no surviving T cells. This ensured that all T cells that developed in the hybrids after this manipulation were derived from the *fresh* bone marrow cells and had matured in the *grafted* thymus.

The fresh bone marrow cells were of the $H-2^{d/k}$ type, but the grafted thymus was $H-2^d$. The question that Zinkernagel was investigating was simply whether the mature T cells from the experimental animals would recognise the MHC molecules encoded by the $H-2^{d/k}$ genes, or only those encoded by $H-2^d$.

☐ Can you suggest a way that he could test for this?

◼ Remember that Zinkernagel (with Peter Doherty) discovered that cytotoxic T cells will only kill virus-infected cells that have self-MHC class I molecules. The question of which MHC molecules are recognised by T cells from the experimental mice can be answered by mixing their T cells with virus-infected cells of three MHC types: $H-2^d$, $H-2^k$ and $H-2^{d/k}$.

When he performed this experiment Zinkernagel found that the T cells could lyse virus-infected cells that carried MHC molecules of the $H-2^d$ or $H-2^{d/k}$ types, but they could not lyse virus-infected $H-2^k$ cells, even though the T cells themselves carried the $H-2^{d/k}$ molecules.

☐ What do you conclude from this?

◼ The T cells were of the $H-2^{d/k}$ type, but they had matured in an $H-2^d$ thymus. The experiment suggests that during their journey through the thymus, the T cells acquired the ability to recognise only the $H-2^d$ molecules that surrounded them. They never acquired the ability to recognise $H-2^k$ molecules, even though these molecules were on the surface of the developing T cells. The crucial point seems to be that $H-2^k$ molecules were *not* on the thymic epithelial cells.

Much more research has been carried out since this experiment caused a stir in immunology, all of which points to the thymus as the source of an 'imprinting' event during T cell development. This results in the mature T cell population becoming committed to recognise antigen only in association with the MHC molecules that occurred on the thymic epithelial cells during T cell maturation. The nature of this 'imprinting' event is still uncertain, but to understand it better we must look more closely at what we mean when we say that 'the T cell population acquired the ability to recognise' certain MHC molecules. This is another way of saying that the emergent T cells have MHC receptors that bind only to certain MHC molecules—in this case the molecules that existed in the thymus—and, conversely, that none of the emergent T cells have MHC receptors that bind to antigen in association with *other* MHC molecules. This doesn't mean that T cells are unresponsive to other MHC molecules. You already know that parts of 'foreign' MHC molecules are recognised as antigens, for example, in transplant rejection. But mature T cells can only recognise 'foreign' MHC *antigens* when they are correctly presented in association with 'self' MHC molecules.

The receptors for 'self' MHC include the CD8 and CD4 molecules, which bind to MHC class I and class II molecules respectively. We know that the long dendritic processes of many thymic epithelial cells are very rich in MHC molecules, and that the developing T cells seem to adhere to these processes as they journey through the thymus. The implication is that those T cells with complementarity between their CD4 or CD8 molecules and the surrounding MHC molecules have a different fate from those that cannot adhere to the thymic epithelial cells as they migrate through the thymus.

Two models for what happens have been proposed. Both assume that thymocytes with a range of *different* CD4 and CD8 molecules are generated by gene recombination during the phase of thymocyte proliferation in the cortex (remember that both these molecules have variable domains; see Figure 4.21). One model proposes that only those thymocytes that have receptors which bind to the MHC molecules of the thymic epithelial cells are selected to develop into mature T cells (**positive thymocyte selection**). Alternatively, thymocytes that have receptors for different MHC molecules from those on thymic cells are destroyed (**negative thymocyte selection**). Dying thymocytes can certainly be detected along the margin between the cortex and the medulla. During this selection process, cells that have *both* CD4 and CD8 also seem to be weeded out, so that the emergent population has one molecule or the other but not both. The signals that trigger development or destruction of thymocytes have not been identified, but thymic epithelial cells produce a range of peptides (known as *thymic hormones*), which are possibly involved.

8.3.2 Generation of T cell antigen receptors

The selection process in the thymus may not end with self-MHC restriction and subset differentiation. T cells also have receptors for epitopes on antigens, and the receptor structures begin to appear quite early in thymocyte development. First, the antigen-specific TcR molecules appear and then, at a later stage, the CD3 chains, which may be involved in signal transduction (see Figure 4.20). Rearrangements of the *VDJ* genes coding for the variable domains of the TcR molecules occur during T cell maturation in the thymus. This results in the generation of clones of mature T cells, each with receptors for a *different* epitope in association with one of the MHC molecules expressed in the individual. During the recombination process, millions of different receptor structures are generated, and it is inevitable that some of them will bind to ligands in molecules that occur *naturally* in the body. In fact, three groups of TcR structures are generated:

(a) TcRs with binding sites for epitopes on foreign antigens;

(b) TcRs with binding sites for *idiotopes*, i.e. for ligands in the structure of secreted or cell-surface antibodies, or in the structure of TcR molecules on other T cells;

(c) TcRs with binding sites for ligands found in molecules on the surface of normal body cells or free in the body fluids.

The function of structures in group (a) is to act as recognition molecules in the immune response to infection; the function of those in group (b) is to regulate the activity of other immune cells (more details are given in Chapter 9); but the structures in group (c) represent a potential threat to the integrity of the body. It is clearly desirable that T cells with antigen receptors for these **self-epitopes** do not participate in damaging immune responses, and most individuals do indeed display **self-tolerance** throughout life. Although the information that we have at present is far from complete, self-tolerance may be due *in part* to a selection process during thymocyte maturation in the thymus, in which T cells with self-reactive TcR structures are suppressed or destroyed. However, this cannot be the whole story. Self-reactive B cells are not all deleted; in fact their existence is quite easy to demonstrate experimentally. And if all self-reactive cells were deleted then the damaging *autoimmune* diseases—in which immune responses are directed against epitopes on naturally occurring molecules in the body—would be extremely rare instead of relatively common. We turn now to the subject of *immunological tolerance*.

8.4   Immunological tolerance

Immunological tolerance refers to the inability of the immune system to react against a particular molecule *even though the immune cells of that individual are capable of generating receptor structures that bind to that molecule*. Under normal circumstances, the immune system of a higher vertebrate is tolerant to all the molecules that occur naturally in its own body (with the exception of idiotopes). But all these molecules are immunogenic if injected into another animal from the same or a different species, so there is nothing intrinsically non-antigenic about their structure. Tolerance can also be induced towards foreign epitopes if the antigen is presented to the immune system early in its development, or if presentation follows certain protocols of dosage and timing. Artificial tolerance induction has shed light on the mechanisms underlying self-tolerance.

8.4.1   The induction of self-tolerance

In the embryo, the precursors of B and T cells are in an immature state. Many experiments have established that they are particularly susceptible to becoming tolerant to any antigen that they meet during this period. The earliest experiment to demonstrate this was performed by R. D. Owen in 1945, who found that non-identical twin cattle would accept skin grafts from each other throughout life if they had shared a placenta during embryonic development (Figure 8.6).

In the 1950s, experiments by Sir Peter Medawar and others established that there is a critical period in the development of the embryo during which self-tolerance is established. Antigens introduced during this period (the duration of which is different for each species) are tolerated throughout life. Figure 8.7 shows the results of one such experiment, in which a mouse from one syngeneic strain was rendered fully tolerant to the cell surface antigens of another mouse strain by injecting cells from a black mouse into the white mouse immediately after birth.

The process by which B cells and T cells become selectively unresponsive to self (or to antigens presented during the critical period) seems to be different for these two cell types.

☐   Suggest three ways in which B cell and T cell tolerance to self-epitopes might be achieved.

■   (a) Selective destruction of any immature B cell that produces surface IgM with binding sites for self-epitopes. (b) Selective destruction of developing helper T cells that have antigen receptors for self-epitopes. (c) Selective activation of suppressor T cells that inhibit immune cells with receptors for self-epitopes.

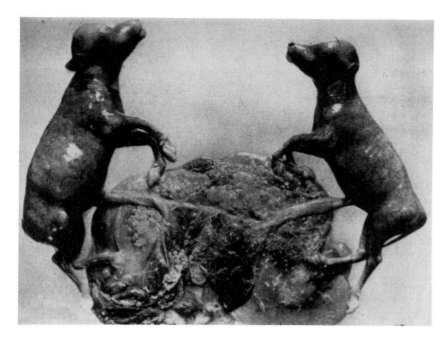

FIGURE 8.6 Non-identical twin cattle fused at the placenta. The blood supply to both embryos is shared, so there is an exchange of cells between them and each remains tolerant to antigens on the other's cells throughout life.

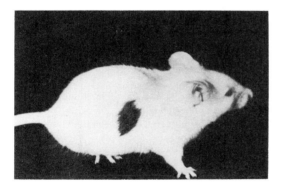

FIGURE 8.7 Tolerance to a foreign skin graft induced by injecting the new-born white mouse with cells from a black mouse. In adult life, the white mouse is fully tolerant to antigens on black mouse cells and will not reject a black skin graft.

These three alternative models of self-tolerance are termed, respectively, **clonal abortion**, **functional deletion** and **T suppression**, and are represented in Figure 8.8.

Clonal abortion of self-reactive B cells was the first model to be proposed and the first to be rejected as a complete explanation. Although some clones of B cells may indeed be deleted in embryonic life, many clones of self-reactive B cells can be detected in adult mammals and birds, but these clones are not normally activated by the self-epitope with which they can react. This points strongly towards the conclusion that self-epitopes behave like T cell-dependent antigens, and that the failure of self-reactive B cell clones to mount an immune response against them must be due to a *lack* of antigen-specific T cell help, to the *presence* of antigen-specific T cell suppression, or to a combination of both.

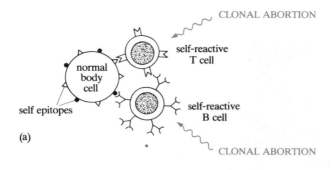

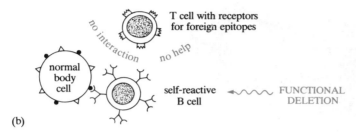

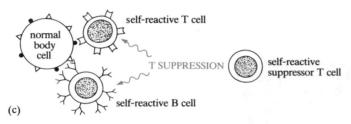

FIGURE 8.8 Theoretical models for the induction and maintenance of self-tolerance: (a) clonal abortion of self-reactive clones of T cells and B cells; (b) functional deletion of surviving self-reactive B cells due to lack of specific T cell help; and (c) suppression of self-reactive clones by specific suppressor T cells.

Most immunologists agree that the primary mechanism of self-tolerance is the absence of antigen-specific T cell help, due to the clonal abortion of many of the relevant clones of anti-self helper T cells during development in the embryo. Suppressor T cells probably act as a back-up by suppressing any self-reactive helper T cell clones that develop in later life, and by direct suppression of the self-reactive B cells.

However, this is an area that contains many unanswered questions. For example, what causes the proposed deletion of these anti-self helper T cell clones? The leading candidate is again the thymus gland, although it may be the *macrophages* and other *antigen-presenting cells* in the thymus rather than the thymic epithelial cells that are involved. It has been proposed that the developing thymocytes which adhere closely to macrophages and APCs in the thymus are destroyed; close adherance suggests a high affinity between the T cell antigen receptor and self-epitopes (in association with MHC molecules) on the surface of the presenting cell.

8.4.2 The artificial induction of tolerance in adult life

There are many situations in which it would be useful to be able to induce tolerance to a particular antigen (or antigens) long after the end of the critical embryonic period in which self-tolerance is established.

☐ Can you suggest some of these situations?

■ Allergy sufferers would benefit from being made tolerant to the allergens that provoke their symptoms; organ and tissue transplantation would be much more successful if complete tolerance to allogeneic MHC molecules could be induced; and diseases caused by autoantibodies might be cured if self-tolerance could be restored.

Although a *general* tolerance to all antigens can be induced by certain drugs, attempts to establish long-lasting tolerance only to *specific* antigens of medical importance have met with little success so far. The problem seems to lie in the nature of the *antigen* to which tolerance is desired, rather than in the ability of the organism to become tolerant. It has proved possible to induce specific tolerance to a great many different antigens in adult experimental rodents, but full tolerance to MHC molecules has only been induced during embryonic life, and this is essential for graft survival.

The experimental induction of tolerance to a specific antigen can be achieved either by repeated injections of very low concentrations of certain weakly immunogenic antigens over a prolonged period (called **low-zone tolerance**), or by giving a single injection of a strongly immunogenic antigen at a very high concentration (**high-zone tolerance**). Low-zone tolerance appears to act solely by activating the clone of suppressor T cells that recognises the antigen, but few antigens can induce it and the tolerance fades quite rapidly. High-zone tolerance is more profound and long lasting because it affects both the T cells and the B cells involved in antigen recognition. The mechanism for inducing high-zone tolerance is not fully understood, but a blockade of all available T cell and B cell receptors by excess antigen seems to be part of the process.

The strategy adopted currently to induce tolerance in human patients results in a generalised immunosuppression. For example, tolerance to allergens is usually achieved by inducing suppressor T cells that inhibit all the B cell clones that produce IgE. Patients with transplants or with autoimmune diseases are usually treated with immunosuppressive drugs that interfere with the ability of cells to divide, and hence inhibit lymphocytes from proliferating after contact with antigen. However, these drugs are toxic to *all* dividing cells (many of them are also used to treat cancers) and they can cause damage to bone marrow and gut cells that have a high turnover. A relatively new drug, *cyclosporin A*, has proved to be much more selective in its effect, and if administered with high doses of the antigen to which tolerance is required, it seems to inhibit only those helper T cell clones that have receptors for that antigen.

8.4.3 The breakdown of self-tolerance

Finally, we turn to the situation in which self-tolerance breaks down. Many **autoimmune diseases** exist in which antibodies and cytotoxic T cells directed against self-epitopes are the primary cause of the pathology (Plate 8.1 illustrates one of them), and **autoantibodies** may aggravate other conditions that are not primarily autoimmune in origin. We review the range of these conditions in the final Chapter of this Book, but for the moment we focus on the mechanisms by which self-tolerance is undermined. Three models have been suggested and are summarised in Figure 8.9.

The first model proposes that new clones of self-reactive helper T cells or B cells may be generated by somatic mutation as an accidental concomitant of the ageing process (Figure 8.9a), and that these clones escape the normal surveillance mechanisms for deleting mutant cells. This model is at least consistent with epidemiological data that show the incidence of autoimmune diseases rising with age. The second model suggests that a *bypass* circuit may develop as a result of a self-epitope becoming modified, say by virus-infection, so that it fits the receptor of a helper T cell. In other words, a T cell receptor that normally binds to a foreign epitope *cross-reacts* with a modified self-epitope. This enables the T cell to activate a pre-existing self-reactive clone of B cells. If you imagine that antigen-specific T cell help requires the T cell and the B cell to be bound simultaneously to the same antigen in close proximity to each other, then you can see from Figure 8.9b how the bypass circuit could operate. The third model proposes that the clone of suppressor T cells responsible for inhibiting the self-reactive T cells or B cells is somehow deleted. All three of these mechanisms may operate in varying degrees in different autoimmune diseases. Whatever the mechanisms, the consequences can be very severe, as you will see in Chapter 10.

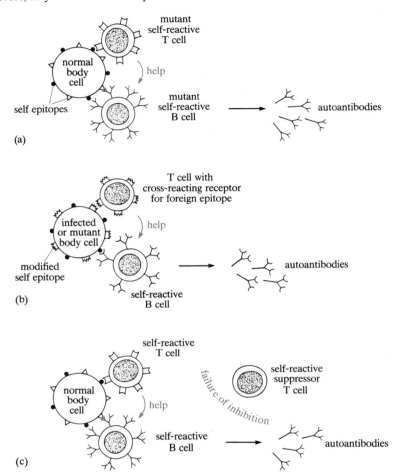

FIGURE 8.9 Theoretical models for the breakdown of self-tolerance: (a) new clones of self-reactive lymphocytes arise by mutation of the antigen-receptor genes; (b) T cells with receptors for foreign epitopes bind to *modified* self-epitopes and this enables them to activate existing clones of self-reactive B cells; and (c) suppressor T cells fail to inhibit self-reactive clones.

Summary of Chapter 8

1   The development of cells involved in adaptive and innate immunity commences early in embryonic life in higher vertebrates, but full immunological competence is not achieved until some time after birth.

2   Immature B cells undergo antigen-independent differentiation into mature B cells in the bone marrow throughout life and in foetal liver. Contact with antigen triggers further differentiation into plasma cells or memory cells. B cell maturation can be traced by the appearance of surface molecules at particular stages of development.

3   Immature T cells (thymocytes) develop in the thymus gland, where clones are selected for maturation or deletion, according to their MHC receptors and antigen receptors, and differentiation into T cell subsets occurs. MHC self-restriction and tolerance to self-epitopes are features of mature T cells. Clonal expansion to active T cells or memory cells follows contact with antigen in association with self-MHC.

4   Tolerance refers to the *inability* of the immune system to direct a damaging immune response against a particular antigen. It depends partly on whether a receptor structure for that antigen exists in the immune system of the individual, and (if it does) on the ability of receptor-binding to trigger a damaging immune response.

5   Self-tolerance, i.e. tolerance to the cells and molecules of the individual's own body, is established during embryonic life and continues into adult life. It results primarily from deletion of self-reactive helper T cells, backed up by the activation of self-reactive suppressor T cells. Tolerance to some antigens (including B cell tolerance) may be artificially induced during adult life if they are administered according to certain protocols.

6   Self-tolerance can break down if new self-reactive clones arise by mutation, if a bypass circuit results from modification of a self-epitope so that it elicits T cell help for self-reactive B cells, or if the inhibitory effect of suppressor T cells is lost.

Now attempt SAQs 30–32, which relate to this Chapter.

CHAPTER 9
REGULATION OF THE IMMUNE RESPONSE

This Chapter is about the ways in which the immune response (adaptive and innate) is regulated. The paramount need for mechanisms that control the onset, magnitude and duration of the immune response must be evident to you from considering the local inflammation and cell death that can characterise the response to an antigen. In this Chapter we briefly describe each of the main regulatory mechanisms (many of which have already been introduced in previous Chapters) and summarise the ways in which they interact. As you study the details of each regulatory mechanism, notice that cell activity is enhanced or inhibited by receptor–ligand interactions at the cell surface. This is the basis of all cell-to-cell communication and the way in which cells detect changes in the concentration of key molecules in their surroundings. The ligand may be an antibody molecule, an antigen, or a cytokine secreted by one of the cells involved in an immune response.

9.1   Regulation by antigen and antibody concentration

The immune response, like many other physiological responses, is subject to regulation by both *positive* and *negative feedback* from changes in the concentration of extracellular ligands. Feedback circuits based on the concentration of *antigen* and the concentration of *antibodies* in the vascular and lymphoid systems illustrate this very well. When a pathogen or parasite first penetrates the physical barriers of the body, the concentration of antigen rises as the infection spreads. This brings the antigen into contact with the receptors of more and more immune cells from the appropriate clones, activating the cells or making them receptive to essential signals from lymphokines synthesised by helper T cells. As antigen concentration falls, owing to the success of the immune response, there is less of it available to activate more immune cells, and the 'driving force' for lymphokine secretion—and hence for B cell stimulation—declines.

Antibody concentration has the opposite effect. As the immune response develops, the concentration of secreted antibodies rises. Initially, the rising concentration of antibodies *enhances* the activity of B cells of the correct clone, so more antibodies are produced. This is one of several *positive* feedback mechanisms in the immune response. But as antigen begins to be eliminated, the output of antibodies 'overshoots' the requirement, and antibodies begin to *inhibit* the activity of B cells once the unbound (i.e. excess) antibody concentration reaches a certain level in the circulation. Immunoglobulins of different classes make different contributions to this feedback circuit: rising levels of free *IgM* are enhancing to B cell activity and precede the class switch to IgG, whereas rising levels of free *IgG* tend to inhibit B cells.

☐ Can you explain the value of the opposite regulatory effects of free IgM and IgG?

■ IgM is secreted at a relatively low concentration mainly during the primary response to an antigen, but the lack of memory cells delays the onset of antibody production; thus, it is useful to have a mechanism for amplifying the response as rapidly as possible once it has begun. In contrast, IgG is produced very quickly and in abundance during the secondary response, owing to the presence of pre-formed memory cells; in this circumstance it is useful to have a mechanism for inhibiting the response once excess IgG is formed.

Excess IgG can inhibit B cells in two ways: it can bind to all the available epitopes on remaining antigens and thus block them from binding to B cells, or it can bind to the Fc receptors on the B cell, which causes inhibition of B cell activity. You may recall from Table 3.1 that B cells have surface receptors for the Fc region of immunoglobulin molecules, and it seems likely that the function of Fc receptors on B cells is to detect excess antibodies and hence regulate the cell's output.

9.2 Regulation by receptor density

The density of receptors on immune cells is not constant and neither is the structure of the receptor. The *density* changes in response to signals received from the surrounding environment, and changes in the structure of expressed receptors can alter the *affinity* of the receptor for the ligand. A striking example of regulation by receptor density involves the receptor for *interleukin-2* (Il-2), a lymphokine secreted by activated helper T cells that recruits other lymphocytes and phagocytes to the immune response (described in Chapter 3; see Table 3.2). Resting T cells (i.e. naive or memory T cells that are *not* in contact with antigen) have no receptors for Il-2, but within a few hours of activation by antigen they begin to transcribe the Il-2 receptor gene, and receptors can be detected on the cell surface within about 24 hours. Activated T cells of the helper subset begin to secrete Il-2, which binds to the Il-2 receptors on nearby T cells and further enhances receptor expression. A positive feedback loop is set up in which the more Il-2 that is bound by a cell, the more the cell expresses Il-2 receptors (Il-2 is *autocrine*, i.e. as well as acting on other cells it is self-stimulating). Moreover, the affinity of the receptors for Il-2 increases as the response proceeds. It has been estimated that active T cells have several thousand high-affinity Il-2 receptors and tens of thousands of low-affinity receptors for this lymphokine. The outcome of Il-2 binding is that the cell is stimulated to proliferate and differentiate into an expanded clone of effector and memory cells.

☐ Il-2 is a *non-specific* stimulator of cell division. How is its effect regulated and focused in an *antigen-specific* way during an immune response?

■ Il-2 receptors are only expressed on T cells *after* contact with antigen, so T cells from clones that are *not* in contact with antigen cannot respond to stimulation by Il-2 in their environment.

The example of Il-2 receptors serves to illustrate a much more widespread phenomenon in which changes in receptor expression regulate aspects of the immune response.

9.3 Regulation by immune cell circuits

We have already set up the basic triad of helper and suppressor T cells acting antagonistically on each other and on effector cells (i.e. cytotoxic T cells, B cells and the cells of innate immunity; see Figure 3.11), but regulatory circuits based on T cells are rather more complex than this. To begin with, the helper T cell subset is not uniform: cells with different functions have been identified within it. For example, some helper cells are involved in the activation of effectors such as B cells and macrophages, whereas others are involved in activating suppressor T cells. Thus, it is possible to divide the helper subset into **inducers of suppression** and **inducers of help** (Figure 9.1) according to whether their activity leads to an amplification or a damping down of the immune response. A further level of control may be contributed by another type of helper cell, termed a **contrasuppressor**, which counteracts the inhibitory effect of suppressor T cells on helper T cells.

There is still considerable uncertainty about whether these regulatory networks are *antigen specific*, in other words, whether the cells in the triad must be in contact with the *same* antigen. Many of the lymphokines that enhance or inhibit the activity of immune cells have been sequenced and their structures are found to be *mono*morphic whatever their source, whereas you would expect them to be *poly*morphic if they were relaying antigen-specific signals. It may be that the regulation of receptor expression on the cells that respond to these lymphokines restricts the responders to a specific clone in close anatomical contact with the originator of the lymphokine (as in the case of Il-2, discussed above), and that this makes the response appear to be antigen specific.

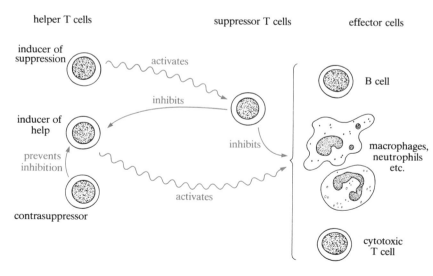

FIGURE 9.1 Regulation of the immune response by networks of T cells. The T cells secrete many types of lymphokine, which have either activating or inhibitory effects on other cells in the immune system.

However, there is evidence in some situations for antigen-specific helper factors or suppressor factors secreted by T cells and acting on other lymphocytes committed to recognise the *same* antigen as the T cell. Antigen-presenting cells are thought to be involved in presenting these factors to the other cells in the circuit, as Figure 9.2 shows. This model predicts the existence of receptors for the helper or suppressor factors on APCs, but evidence for their existence is not conclusive.

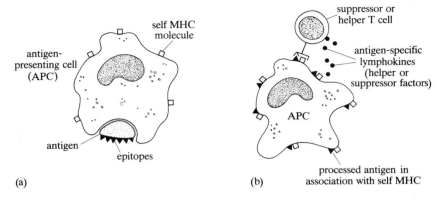

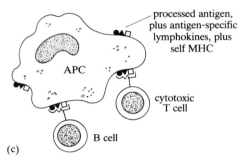

FIGURE 9.2 A theoretical role for antigen-presenting cells (APCs) in antigen-specific regulation of T and B cell activity. (a) Antigen is engulfed and processed by the APC; (b) antigen-specific helper or suppressor factors are released by T cells in contact with the processed antigen and MHC molecules at the APC surface; and (c) the suppressor or helper factors are presented by the APC to other immune cells that have receptors for the same antigen.

Yet another regulatory circuit exists, which involves all types of lymphocytes, is independent of antigen, and is based on the fact that parts of the antigen receptors of T cells and B cells are themselves immunogenic. This type of regulation is mediated through *idiotype networks*.

9.3.1 Idiotype network regulation

Several times in this Book we have mentioned the fact that with at least 10^8 different receptor structures in the immune system it would be surprising if some of these polypeptides were not mutually interactive. The variable domains of immunoglobulins and T cell antigen receptors contain clusters of residues that are immunogenic in the originating animal. Each of these clusters is called an **idiotope**, and molecules that include idiotopes in their structure are called **idiotypes** (i.e. an idiotype is a specific arrangement of idiotopes on the same molecule; see Figure 9.3a). Some idiotopes are unique to a particular molecular structure (i.e. they occur on a specific idiotype and nowhere else) and these are termed **private idiotopes**; by contrast, **public idiotopes** have a more widespread distribution and occur on many different idiotypes. Inevitably, the private idiotopes are most likely to be found in the hypervariable parts of recognition molecules, for example, in the binding sites for antigen (Figure 9.3b).

Some clones of helper and suppressor T cells have receptors with binding sites for particular idiotopes, and some clones of B cells synthesise antibodies with binding sites for idiotopes. These receptor or antibody molecules are termed **anti-idiotypes** (Figure 9.4). Notice from Figure 9.4 that if the *idiotope* is part of the binding site for antigen, then the *anti-idiotype* that binds with it may *resemble* the antigen in its shape. Anti-idiotypes that fit into the binding site for antigen are referred to as carrying an **internal image** of the antigen.

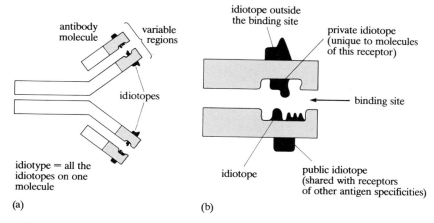

FIGURE 9.3 (a) Together all the *idiotopes* on a receptor molecule constitute an *idiotype* (the antibody molecule shown here could be replaced by a T cell antigen receptor). (b) Close-up view of an antigen binding site on an antibody molecule or T cell receptor. *Private* idiotopes are unique to a particular idiotype and are therefore often in the binding site; *public* idiotopes are found on several different idiotypes.

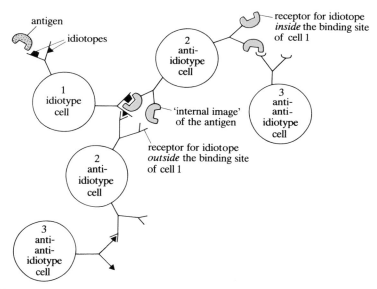

FIGURE 9.4 Idiotype/anti-idiotype regulation by networks of helper and suppressor cells. The helper and suppressor cells have receptors for idiotopes that are inside or on the outside of the binding site on the antigen receptors of other cells in the network. Level 1 cells have receptors for a particular antigen, but idiotopes on these receptors are bound by receptors on level 2 cells, some of which *resemble* the antigen (these are the 'internal image' receptors). Idiotopes on the level 2 receptors are, in turn, bound by receptors on level 3 cells, and further levels may exist. Interactions between receptors via idiotype/anti-idiotype interactions may either activate or inhibit cells in the network in the *absence* of antigen.

☐ What do you think might happen if an internal image anti-idiotype bound to the antigen receptor of a helper T cell?

■ It might have the same effect as antigen binding, i.e. it might activate the T cell without the need for antigen.

☐ Suppose that a large number of identical anti-idiotypes bound to a certain public idiotope wherever it occurred in the immune system. What effect might this have?

■ A large number of different lymphocyte clones would be affected (regardless of their antigen specificity) because this idiotope is common to all of them somewhere in their receptor structures. The location of the idiotope on the receptor structure would determine whether the clones were activated or inhibited by interaction with anti-idiotype.

But it does not stop there! The anti-idiotype molecules themselves have idiotopes that are recognised by other clones of T cells and B cells, which have receptors known as **anti-anti-idiotypes** on their surfaces (also shown in Figure 9.4).

The Norwegian immunologist Niels Jerne proposed in 1974 that a network of regulatory circuits based on idiotype/anti-idiotype/anti-anti-idiotype interactions existed independently of antigen. At the time it was a controversial proposition, but evidence for the existence of **idiotype network regulation** is now conclusive, although many of the details remain to be elucidated. Jerne was awarded a Nobel prize in 1984 (shared with Milstein and Köhler; see Chapter 7) for his extensive and varied contributions to immunological knowledge, of which idiotype networks are just a part. The network is thought to operate broadly as follows. B cells can be activated *without the need for antigen* if their antigen receptors are cross-linked by anti-idiotypes. (This is exactly analogous to the activation of B cells when their antigen receptors are cross-linked by repeating polymer antigens, illustrated in Figure 3.6a. Cross-linking of membrane-bound receptors seems to be one of several devices for transmitting signals across the cell membrane.) In addition, helper and suppressor T cells whose receptors are anti-idiotypes may activate or inhibit B cells and other T cells directly (without antigen) by binding to their idiotopes (Figure 9.5).

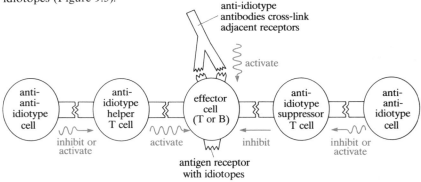

FIGURE 9.5 One model of how idiotype network regulation may operate. Effector cells may be activated (in the absence of antigen) either by anti-idiotype antibodies, which cross-link B cell receptors by binding to idiotopes, or by anti-idiotype helper T cells. Suppression is mediated by anti-idiotype suppressor T cells. A further level of regulation may be provided by anti-anti-idiotype helper or suppressor cells, which activate or inhibit other members of the network.

The activity of anti-idiotype clones is further regulated by anti-anti-idiotype clones, and so on. No one is quite sure how many levels of regulation exist, and opinion is divided on how important idiotype networks are in relation to the lymphokine-mediated regulatory circuits discussed earlier. Jerne proposed that the idiotype networks have a special role in maintaining self-tolerance by holding the immune system in a suppressed state with respect to self-epitopes. Interactions between idiotype regulation and lymphokine regulation must contribute to the overall fine-tuning of the immune response to external antigens.

9.4 Genetic control of immune responsiveness

The mechanisms by which immune regulation is achieved operate within genetic constraints that are unique to each individual. The extent of the immune response to the *same* antigen differs between non-identical individuals of the same species.

Some individuals will respond very powerfully to a particular antigen, others only moderately and some may not respond to it at all. These differences are measures of the **immune responsiveness** of each individual to a particular antigen. Moreover, antigens that provoke a high response in one individual may provoke a low response in someone else, so each individual has a particular immune responsiveness *pattern* characterised by precisely which antigens are responded to and in what degree.

The extent of an individual's immune responsiveness to different antigens is determined in part by which alleles they express in certain regions of the *major histocompatibility complex* (*MHC*). If you look back at Figure 4.18 you will see the relative positions of the genes of the *MHC* in the human and in the mouse genome. Experiments with congenic strains of mice have shown that the combination of alleles found in the *I region* of the mouse *MHC* has a significant effect on the ability of the mouse to mount an immune response to particular antigens. A change of allele at either the *IA* or *IE* locus is enough to convert a strain from being a low responder to a high responder (or vice versa) for a given antigen. This has led to the genes in the *I region* being referred to as **immune responsiveness genes**, or **Ir genes** for short. Notice that genes in this region also code for class II MHC molecules.

☐ Explain how the class II molecules could be involved in immune responsiveness.

■ These molecules include binding sites for processed antigen, which is then recognised in association with the class II molecules by helper T cells. It is logical to conclude that the structure of the class II molecules determines how well the molecule will associate with a particular antigen, and this in turn affects how well the antigen can be presented to helper T cells. 'Poor' presentation leads to a low response.

The class I molecules are also involved in immune responsiveness in a number of ways. They not only associate with antigen and enable its correct presentation to cytotoxic T cells, but they also associate with many different receptors in the surface membrane of the cell on which they are expressed. For example, the extent to which the class I molecules associate with Il-2 receptors in the membrane of activated T cells alters the *affinity* of the receptor for Il-2, and hence the responsiveness of the cell to this lymphokine. Class I molecules have also been found in association with receptors for insulin and epidermal growth factor, altering ligand-binding to these receptors. Remember that class I molecules are found on virtually every cell in the body, so they may have a widespread modulating effect on cell-to-cell interactions, beyond their role in immune responsiveness.

Genetic restrictions on the activity and interactions of immune cells have been demonstrated in many different ways in mice, and all these effects map to the *MHC* genes. For example, it has been demonstrated in mice that T cell help is only available to B cells that have the same alleles in the *I region*. The effect of particular alleles at particular loci in the *MHC* genes has been mapped more extensively in mice than in humans, but all the evidence shows that the *HLA complex* in humans is exactly homologous to the *H-2 complex* in mice. The *D region* of the human *HLA* genes has similar properties to the *I region* of mouse *H-2*, i.e. the alleles found at the *DP*, *DQ* and *DR* loci have a central role in determining immune responsiveness. Furthermore, genes *outside* the *MHC* in both species also influence immune responsiveness, although the effects of these genes are generalised rather than antigen specific. For example, they restrict the production of complement components. Thus, the immune response is regulated in part by genetically determined restrictions on the *structure* of receptor molecules on immune cells, and on the level of *responsiveness* and *cooperation* between immune cells. As you will see in Chapter 10, these genetic restrictions have implications for the susceptibility of the individual to particular infections and to certain non-infectious diseases, especially those with an autoimmune component.

9.5 Regulation by neuroendocrine mechanisms

We conclude this discussion by mentioning an area of increasing research activity: interactions between the immune system, the nervous system and the endocrine system in regulating the internal environment. Although our focus here is on the ways in which neuroendocrine mechanisms exert control over the immune response, it is important to recognise that the level of activity of the immune system also exerts an effect on the activity of the nervous system and on certain endocrine glands. The communication is two-way. Much remains to be discovered about these interactions and much has been speculated about their significance.

The starting point for this discussion must be to emphasise that all the primary and secondary lymphoid organs are innervated, and that lymphocytes have receptors for a number of neurotransmitter substances and hormones. Moreover, most neurons in the peripheral and central nervous system have surface molecules that are also found on certain subsets of immune cells, and that are structurally related to the immunoglobulins (for example, the molecule known as Thy-1; see Figure 4.21). Although the function of most of these shared molecules is unknown, their existence strongly suggests that neurons and immune cells communicate with each other by the transfer of chemical signals.

The extent of the influence of neuroendocrine regulation on the activity of the immune system can be demonstrated very strikingly by classical Pavlovian conditioning experiments. (In the first experiment of this type, Pavlov was able to condition dogs to salivate when a bell was rung. He did this by associating the sound with the arrival of food on a number of occasions, until the bell alone would elicit the conditioned response.) It has proved possible to condition mice to suppress their own immune responses. One experiment used a particular strain of mice that spontaneously develop an autoimmune disease, which can be reversed by administering immunosuppressive drugs. If the drug is given in association with a conditioning stimulus, such as ringing a bell, then the mice can be maintained in a disease-free state by regular exposure to the conditioning stimulus *without* the drug. In a similar vein, much publicity has been given to experiments on the use of hypnosis in human subjects to prolong the survival of foreign skin grafts.

The mechanisms that mediate these effects are unknown. However, it is known that lesions in certain regions of the brain can induce either immunosuppression or enhancement of the immune response, and the electrical stimulation of lymphoid organs by excitatory or inhibitory neurons can make lymphocytes more susceptible or more refractory to stimulation by antigen or lymphokines. Moreover, the output of all endocrine (hormone-secreting) glands is ultimately influenced by the nervous system, either by direct innervation of the gland or through releasing factors secreted by the hypothalamus. Lymphocytes have receptors for a number of hormones, particularly those involved in the so-called **adrenal axis** (Figure 9.6). In brief, this axis consists of the pituitary gland, which secretes adrenocorticotropic hormone (ACTH), which stimulates the adrenal gland to secrete a range of hormones collectively known as glucocorticoids. The glucocorticoids are immunosuppressive. They exert their effect by inhibiting the synthesis of interleukin-1 by macrophages and the synthesis of lymphokines by helper T cells.

The adrenal axis is not the only contributor to endocrine regulation of the immune response. Other hormones are also immunosuppressive, for example, insulin and some of the sex hormones (androgens, oestrogens and progestogens); whereas growth hormone, thyroid hormone and oxytocin have enhancing effects on certain elements of the immune response, particularly the cytotoxic activity of NK cells. The many complex interactions between the immune system, the nervous system and the endocrine system have led to the notion that immune cells are in part an information-gathering network for the brain, transmitting information back about the extent to which pathogens have infected the body, and recruiting assistance from neuroendocrine regulatory circuits.

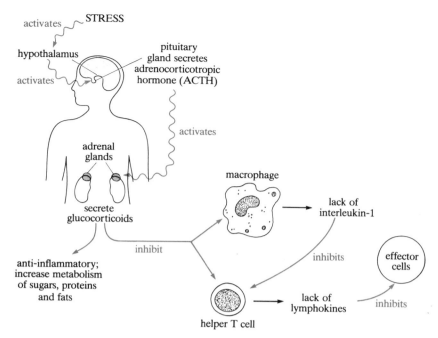

FIGURE 9.6 The adrenal axis links the hypothalamus to the secretion of glucocorticoid hormones by the adrenal glands. Activation of the adrenal axis (for example, by stress) leads to a generalised immunosuppression mediated by glucucorticoids, which inhibit the activity of macrophages and helper T cells.

However, there are certain flaws in the reasoning underlying this attractive hypothesis. Infectious illness is stressful, so you might predict that stress should *enhance* immune responsiveness through neuroendocrine activity. In fact, the opposite appears to be the case. The adrenal axis is activated by stress (a notoriously difficult concept to define—a task we shall not attempt here), and this has led to a number of experiments demonstrating that stressful procedures such as electric shocks induce immunosuppression. Stress also causes the release of peptides that resemble derivatives of opium from neurons in the brain, and these *endorphins* have immunosuppressive effects as well as altering pain perception. A number of investigations of human subjects in stressful situations (for example, after bereavement or during university examinations) have shown that certain elements of their immune response are *less* effective than those of controls.

It is difficult to demonstrate conclusively that stress-related immunosuppression has health consequences, although athletes in intensive training have been shown to be significantly more susceptible to infection than fit adults who are not undertaking strenuous exercise. We know that immune responsiveness fluctuates under neuroendocrine influence according to *diurnal* and *circadian* rhythms; it may be that the normal variations from day to day or from season to season are no greater than the variations observed in putatively stressful and non-stressful situations. Nevertheless, advocates of the newly-popular research into psycho-neuroimmunology are convinced that emotional state can influence health through neuroendocrine regulation of the immune system.

Summary of Chapter 9

1   The concentration of free antigen and free antibodies in the circulation has an enhancing effect early in the immune response, and an inhibitory effect later in the response.

2   Circuits of helper and suppressor T cells exist that are able to amplify or inhibit the immune response to a particular antigen by secreting certain lymphokines and

(possibly) antigen-specific helper of suppressor factors. Regulation is achieved in part by changes in density and affinity of receptors for these signalling molecules.

3   The activity of immune cells is further regulated, independently of antigen, by networks of T cells and B cells with receptors for immunogenic idiotopes that are on the antigen receptors of lymphocytes of all subsets and antigen specificities. Idiotype/anti-idiotype interactions can either activate or inhibit immune cells, and are themselves subject to further levels of control by anti-anti-idiotypes.

4   Genetic restrictions on the structure and expression of receptors involved in immune interactions regulate the level of immune responsiveness to each antigen and the extent of cell-to-cell communication.

5   Interactions between cells in the immune, nervous and endocrine systems contribute to the regulation of the immune response, but the regulatory mechanisms are far from fully understood.

Now attempt SAQs 33–35, which relate to this Chapter.

CHAPTER 10
DISORDERS OF IMMUNITY

In the final Chapter in this Book, we consider the most common disorders of the immune system and the mechanisms by which they produce their characteristic symptoms. We aim to give you a basic understanding of the immune disfunctions underlying these disorders because they are responsible for considerable human suffering, and also because they provide compelling illustrations of what happens when the normal interaction and regulation of immune cells and their products breaks down.

10.1   Immunopathology

Immunopathology refers to disease states that arise primarily from the action or inaction of immune mechanisms. Immune disorders can be divided into those that result from immune *deficiency*, and those that result from immune *hyperactivity* of one or more elements of the immune response, including responses directed against inappropriate targets. This is the way that we have chosen to discuss this subject, but you should recognise that an alternative way of categorising immunopathology is to look at what *causes* the hyperactivity or deficiency state to arise. The problem with this method is that so many immune disorders, including most of the autoimmune diseases and cancers originating from immune cells, are of unknown cause.

However, in the discussion that follows, look out for what evidence there is about causes. For example, immune deficiency or hyperactivity states can be provoked by external agents such as pathogens and allergens, or by the medical use of radiation or drugs (the states may be *iatrogenic*, i.e. caused by medical intervention). Immunopathology can also be *idiopathic* (i.e. spontaneously arising without any known external provocation). The influence of genetic factors can be detected in both deficiency and hyperactivity disorders. For example, many spontaneous deficiency disorders are apparent from birth or arise during development only in people who have a particular genetic constitution, and some autoimmune diseases also show an association with certain alleles in the genes of the major histocompatibility complex (*MHC*). And since there is a genetic component to immune responsiveness, it is also reasonable to conclude that there is a genetic contribution to each person's ability to resist infectious disease.

10.2 Congenital immune deficiency

Heritable disorders of the immune system are rare and almost all result in **congenital immune deficiency** rather than hyperactivity. The pattern of disorders that arise from the primary deficiency is determined by which element of the immune system is absent or defective. You may recall the earlier discussion of congenital immune deficiencies affecting either B cell or T cell development (Chapters 2 and 3).

☐ What are the general differences in susceptibility to different types of pathogens between people with B cell deficiencies and those with T cell deficiencies?

■ Very broadly, people with B cell deficiencies are more prone to bacterial infections but have relatively normal resistance to viral infections. People with T cell deficiencies show the opposite pattern of susceptibility, unless they have total T cell loss (as in children born without a thymus gland), which results in profound susceptibility to most pathogens.

B cell deficiencies are by far the most common congenital immune disorder, and several types are more common in males than in females owing to linkage of recessive traits with the X-chromosome. Other heritable immune deficiencies have been identified in which phagocytic cells have a metabolic defect that prevents them from generating one or other of the degradative enzymes or oxidising agents in the lysosomes, or that prevents fusion of the lysosome with the vacuole surrounding the engulfed pathogen. The result is that intracellular pathogens thrive inside the phagocyte, and in severe cases this may prove fatal to the person.

Genetically determined *complement* deficiencies, though extremely rare, are as varied as the many functions associated with the different serum proteins of this complex system. Deficiency of components that act as opsonins (e.g. C3b) greatly reduces the effectiveness of phagocytic cells. This leads to disorders resulting from the failure to eliminate immune complexes, or to life-threatening infections, particularly from the bacteria causing pneumonia, meningitis and peritonitis.

10.3 Induced immunosuppression

Otherwise healthy individuals may become **immunosuppressed** as a result of the action of certain external agents, which interfere with the normal ability of cells in the immune system to proliferate or to differentiate into effector cells. Whatever the cause, the consequence is that the person may become susceptible to a range of infections that would normally be eliminated by the immune response. Infectious diseases that result in severe, even fatal, illness in an immunosuppressed person but not in an immunocompetent person are known collectively as **opportunistic infections**, and they include several pathogens that normally only affect other species. We will briefly review the external agents that can induce immunosuppression, ending with the most topical—the virus that can lead to AIDS.

10.3.1 Ionising radiation and immunosuppressive drugs

Bone marrow is very sensitive to ionising radiation (X-rays and the sort emitted by radioactive isotopes) because the cells are rapidly dividing. Immunosuppression can be induced by giving whole-body irradiation of a very carefully controlled dosage, which destroys the stem cells from which all blood cells are derived. This is a high-risk procedure because radiation causes damage to many other tissues, particularly in the lungs and gut, but it is performed in cases where a complete replacement of a person's bone marrow is necessitated by a cancer of the white cells. Partial immunosuppression is an unavoidable side-effect of the localised radiation used to treat many cancers, and is also one of many life-threatening consequences of accidental exposure to radiation.

Immunosuppression is induced by certain drugs in patients who are the recipients of tissue or organ grafts from a non-identical individual, and it is also an option in the treatment of severe immune hyperactivity disorders, such as allergies or autoimmune diseases. A mild immunosuppression can be induced by administering glucocorticoids (see Figure 9.6), but this is not adequate to preserve a foreign graft or to control many autoimmune diseases. A profound generalised immunosuppression can be induced by drugs that interfere with nucleic acid synthesis, which therefore mainly affect rapidly dividing cells, such as cancers, bone-marrow stem cells and lymphocytes stimulated by antigen. This strategy inevitably leaves the patient susceptible to a wide range of infections. However, in the 1970s a new drug, *cyclosporin A*, was introduced and this has greatly improved the success of transplants by inducing a far more specific immunosuppression. It is thought to interfere with the translation of mRNA into lymphokines, and also to inhibit the expression of receptors for Il-2 on T cells and B cells. It is taken up only by T cells and B cells that are in the earliest phase of mitosis.

☐ How does this produce a more graft-specific immunosuppression in a transplant patient, and why is this preferable for the patient?

■ In a patient who has just received an organ transplant, most of the *newly activated* lymphocytes will be responding to antigens on the graft. These cells are rendered ineffective by the drug because they are prevented from expressing Il-2 receptors or from secreting certain lymphokines, and hence from participating in the immune response. But *quiescent* memory T cells and B cells are not affected, so immune responsiveness to most pathogens is preserved.

The goal for the future is to induce an antigen-specific immunosuppression, but human organ transplants present the recipient's immune system with many different epitopes (mainly products of the donor's *MHC* genes), so it is perhaps too ambitious to hope that a specific suppression of all the clones that recognise those epitopes will be achieved. Some initial success has already been reported in experimental animals injected with monoclonal antibodies directed against private (unique) idiotopes on the antigen receptors of lymphocytes that bind to the graft. A related strategy is to inject the idiotopes themselves, attached to a suitable carrier, and thereby induce suppressive anti-idiotype antibodies in the recipient.

10.3.2 Parasite-induced immunosuppression

Of the many escape mechanisms possessed by parasites, induced immunosuppression is the most widespread strategy. Chemical compounds secreted by many types of parasite directly inhibit the activity of B cells, macrophages or cytotoxic T cells. In a few cases they also induce the proliferation of suppressor T cells that specifically inhibit effector cells directed against the parasite. An alternative means of inducing immunosuppression is by exhausting the immune response either by the polyclonal activation of B cells, or by flooding the circulation with so much antigen that all available receptors are blocked or high-zone tolerance is induced. The success of these immunosuppressive strategies in preserving parasites inside their hosts, in some cases indefinitely, is testified by the appalling numbers of people affected by parasitic infestations—at least two thousand million worldwide.

10.3.3 Human immunodeficiency virus (HIV)

The underlying cause of **acquired immune deficiency syndrome (AIDS)** is a virus that, after some dispute, has been given the internationally agreed title of **human immunodeficiency virus**, or **HIV**. HIV is a **retrovirus**, that is, it has RNA, not DNA, as its genetic material. After infecting a cell, the viral RNA is transcribed into DNA using the enzyme *reverse transcriptase*, and the viral DNA is then spliced into the genome of the infected cell and is later expressed in the manufacture of new virus particles. HIV also belongs to a retrovirus subgroup known as the *lentiviruses* (from the Latin *lentus* meaning slow), so named because several years may pass before symptoms develop in an infected person.

After a highly variable incubation period, HIV induces a profound immunosuppression which renders the infected person susceptible to numerous opportunistic infections and one epithelial cell cancer. HIV infects only those cells in the body that have surface-bound CD4 molecules, because the virus particles have receptors that bind only to CD4, and receptor binding is essential before the viral RNA can be incorporated into the cell. CD4 molecules are found abundantly on all mature helper T cells and, in much lower density, on the surface of tissue macrophages and antigen-presenting cells in various sites, perhaps most importantly in the brain. The viral genome is incorporated into the genetic material of the host cell and may remain 'dormant' there for several years. The trigger for expression of the viral genome may be when the cell is activated by contact with the antigen for which it has receptors. Helper T cells in which the viral genome is being expressed become factories for new virus particles, and cell death results as thousands of new particles are shed from the infected cell (Figure 10.1). Some of these infected cells may also be killed by cytotoxic T cells with receptors for HIV antigens. The helper:suppressor ratio begins to fall as helper T cells die, and this shift can often be detected before the onset of disease symptoms. The number of helper T cells continues to fall and they may disappear altogether from the peripheral circulation in severely affected people. Inevitably, the ability of the person to respond to new antigens declines with the collapse of the helper T cell population.

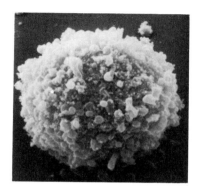

FIGURE 10.1 Scanning electron microscope photograph of a helper T cell infected with human immunodeficiency virus (HIV), magnified 7 500 times. Thousands of small spherical virus particles can be seen 'budding' from the ruffled surface of the cell. As they are released the cell is destroyed.

It is interesting to note that immunity to infections from which the person has recovered prior to contact with HIV remains more or less intact. This is because memory cells (like suppressor T cells) are resistant to the virus, and HIV-infected macrophages and other types of antigen-presenting cell are *not* killed by the replicating viruses that they harbour. The B cells in AIDS patients also seem to be *polyclonally* activated because unusually large amounts of circulating antibodies to a great many antigens are found in their serum, apparently in the absence of stimulation by those antigens.

Infection with HIV has a very variable outcome. At one end of the spectrum are people who have survived without symptoms for seven or eight years, and who have not become immunosuppressed. At the other end of the spectrum is full-blown AIDS, which has so far been fatal in all patients within two years of diagnosis. In between these extremes are people experiencing episodes of milder HIV-related illness interspersed with periods of recovery. Very little is understood about why there is such a variation in the degree of immunosuppression induced by HIV, or why some people remain disease-free for a long time and then suddenly become ill.

AIDS is termed a deficiency *syndrome* because the symptoms vary from patient to patient. Symptoms depend on which pathogens colonise the infected person, whether or not the brain is affected, and whether the patient develops an otherwise rare cancer of blood vessel tissue, known as *Kaposi sarcoma*, which is a particularly common feature of AIDS. AIDS patients characteristically suffer from severe episodes of pneumonia, night sweats and fevers, swollen lymph nodes, diarrhoea and weight loss caused by opportunistic infections. *Pneumocystis carinii*, an organism that resembles a protozoon but which shows a closer genetic relationship to fungi, is particularly common. It infects the lungs and causes an intractable pneumonia. Other complications involve the spread of HIV or opportunistic infections to the brain and spinal cord, which can result in mood-swings, fits, loss of motor coordination and memory, dementia and, occasionally, brain tumours.

At the time of writing (1989), a great deal of research activity is in progress aimed at developing a vaccine to protect people against infection with HIV, but success seems a long way off. People who have been infected with HIV readily produce antibodies that bind to epitopes on the virus, but these antibodies are not protective and have no apparent effect on the ability of the virus to bind to and invade host cells. The other mechanisms by which the immune response normally controls viruses (cytotoxic T cells, NK activity and interferon) are also unable to prevent HIV from gaining a hold on the helper T cell population. The most effective strategy currently available to control the spread of infection in the population is to alter the behaviours that place people at risk.

HIV is transmitted only by direct transfer of infected blood or semen (and possibly breast milk) from person to person. This is most likely to occur during sexual intercourse and artificial insemination; during blood transfusion, the injection of Factor VIII prepared from unscreened blood (to treat haemophilia) and other invasive medical, surgical and dental procedures; through the injection of drugs using contaminated needles or syringes; by transfer from mother to foetus during pregnancy or at childbirth, and possibly through breast feeding. There are a very few cases in which infection has resulted from blood being splashed on to broken skin or from needle-stick injuries (accidental jabs) sustained by health care workers mishandling medical 'sharps' after treating AIDS patients. There is no evidence that HIV can be transmitted in saliva, sweat or tears, or by non-sexual physical contact, even though virus particles can be detected in some of these body fluids.

The reason for the high infectivity of blood and semen and the non-infectivity of saliva is thought to reflect the requirement either for large volumes of 'free' virus particles to be transferred (as in blood transfusions or Factor VIII) or for infected lymphocytes or macrophages to be transferred from person to person. This could explain why semen is generally so infective, since it contains many macrophages, whereas saliva contains few, if any, and it also contains an enzyme that inactivates the virus. However, there are a number of well documented cases of the regular sexual partners of infected people remaining uninfected with HIV despite several years of exposure. Infectivity seems to depend partly on the output of virus or virus-infected cells by the infected person, and partly on the susceptibility of their partner to infection. The idea of a 'critical dose' of virus as one requirement for infection may also explain why accidental needle-stick injuries have such a low infectivity (only four people in over 1 000 documented accidents had formed antibodies to HIV by the beginning of 1989), whereas injecting drug users who share needles and syringes run a high risk of infection. Needle-sticks tend to be superficial jabs which are not repeated, whereas drug users tend to inject themselves deeply and repeatedly, and often flush the syringe with blood to withdraw residual drops of the drug.

While there is little progress to report in the development of new drugs or vaccines that might halt the spread of HIV in the population, it is worth reinforcing the message that for most people in the industrialised world it is an entirely avoidable infection. Blood and blood products are screened, so transmission is now restricted to sexual or drug-related behaviours. Although the epidemic was initially confined to homosexual men in the USA, it has now spread far beyond the gay community, and the exponential increase in the incidence of AIDS among heterosexuals— particularly in central and eastern African countries—may pose the most serious threat to human health on a global scale since the plague pandemics of the Middle Ages.

10.4 Cancers: immune deficiency or immune hyperactivity?

Cancers have often been represented as immune deficiency disorders, and occasionally as a consequence of immune hyperactivity. We have mentioned cancers at very few points in the preceding Chapters. This may have surprised you because there has been a great deal of publicity for the idea that the immune system is 'on surveillance' for malignant cells as well as for pathogens and other external antigens. From this viewpoint, cancers could be seen as arising from the inability of the immune response to eliminate them—in other words, as the consequence of an immune deficiency.

However, there is a serious flaw in this reasoning. In order for the immune system to detect them, malignant cells must have surface properties that differ from the surface membranes of normal cells, and lymphocytes, macrophages and the other contributors to the immune response must have receptors that bind specifically to tumour cells. Although tumour-specific antigens have been demonstrated on artificially induced mouse tumour cells, it has transpired that almost all of them are either retrovirus proteins (inbred laboratory mice are hosts for many such viruses), or they are found only on tumours induced by powerful carcinogenic chemicals administered to the mice. Spontaneously arising cancers in mice, like those in humans, do not have tumour-specific antigens. Attempts to influence the progression of spontaneous cancers by manipulating the immune response have been disappointing, and in some cases have resulted in *accelerated* tumour progression. Despite many years of hopeful research and speculation, general theories of immune surveillance against cancers have collapsed. A key finding that undermined the theory was that the rate of spontaneous cancers is normal in a strain of inbred mouse that has no thymus gland, and hence no functional adaptive immunity (they are called *nude* mice because they have no hair).

☐ Can you think of a disease state in which you would expect cancers to proliferate if they were really under immune surveillance?

■ AIDS patients should, in theory, be prone to many cancers. In reality they are prone only to one (Kaposi sarcoma) that is not explained by infection.

However, the fact that Kaposi sarcoma proliferates in immunosuppressed people suggests that this cancer *is* normally under immune control; the mechanisms are poorly understood, but probably involve tissue macrophages. It may be that some other epithelial-cell or skin-cell cancers are also controlled by innate mechanisms. However, one or two of these are caused by viruses, so in these cases the immune response is recognising viral rather than tumour-specific antigens. Very few of the major fatal cancers are thought to involve viruses as part of their causal mechanisms, but there is scope for influencing the progression of those that do by manipulating the immune response.

There are other ways in which **immunotherapy** may play a part in the treatment of cancers. The cells of most spontaneous solid-tissue cancers (i.e. all cancers except the leukaemias and lymphomas that originate in the immune system) can be shown to have membrane-bound peptides that are normally found only on embryonic cells. These molecules are not immunogenic in the animal bearing the tumour because they were present during its earlier development, but they nevertheless distinguish normal adult body cells from malignant cells. It has proved possible to elicit antibodies to these molecules by injecting them into other individuals or species, which respond to them as antigens. These molecules have therefore been termed **onco-foetal antigens** (*oncos* is Greek for 'lump'). You have already been introduced to one of these molecules, carcinoembryonic antigen, which is a member of the immunoglobulin supergene family (see Figure 4.21 and the discussion of embryonic antigens in section 6.4.3). Monoclonal antibodies directed against onco-foetal antigens have been synthesised, and some limited success has been achieved in targeting low-energy radioactive molecules on to cancers for diagnostic purposes (as discussed in Chapter 7). The hope for the future is to use antibodies directed against these molecules as carriers for highly toxic molecules that will kill the malignant cells.

Investigation of the genes that code for onco-foetal antigens has led to a fundamental re-thinking by biologists of the way in which the malignant state is viewed. Cancer cells are no longer likened to a foreign tissue graft, but are seen as cells that have regained or retained properties that are appropriately expressed only during embryonic development. Cancer cells express genes that should normally be repressed in adult life. Thus cancer cells, like embryonic cells, are relatively unspecialised and undifferentiated, proliferate very rapidly, may move around the body to take up new locations and are not immobilised by contact with nearby cells. The genes that are inappropriately activated in malignant cells have been termed **oncogenes**. There was confusion for a time about whether these oncogenes had originated in viruses, because almost identical genes were sequenced from a few virus strains that were able to induce cancers in experimental animals. Current wisdom agrees that the direction of gene transfer has in fact been the other way: the oncogenic viruses are thought to have acquired their oncogenes from the genome of host cells that they infected at some point in evolution.

To sum up, the major fatal cancers of the lung, gut, breast and urinogenital tract proliferate without check from the immune system because the cells of these cancers are not immunogenic, and *not* because the immune system is deficient. The normal incidence of the major solid cancers in transplant patients who have been immunosuppressed for long periods is further confirmation that immune surveillance against most kinds of malignant cells is at most a minor activity of the immune system. However, transplant patients do suffer from a significant increase in the incidence of cancers originating in leukocytes. The most likely explanation for the raised numbers of leukaemias, lymphomas and myelomas in transplant patients is that the drugs used to suppress immune cells are also carcinogenic to them.

Cancers of the immune system itself are relatively common in the general population and could be viewed as disorders of immune hyperactivity. Under normal circumstances, immune cells remain quiescent for long periods but then switch into a period of rapid and exponential proliferation after contact with antigen. The genes underlying this proliferative activity can become permanently expressed if they are transferred to a different part of the genome, away from the regulator sequences that normally keep them repressed. Translocation of particular gene sequences is very commonly found in leukaemias and lymphomas. For example, the gene known as *c-myc* (which is involved in precipitating the start of mitosis), the B cell immunoglobulin genes, and the T cell receptor genes are frequently found in unusual locations in the cells of these cancers. One hope for cancer research of the future is to find ways of correcting the effects of these translocations and of regulating the expression of oncogenes, rather than to discover drugs that kill cancer cells.

We turn now to non-malignant states of *immune hyperactivity*, characterised by the inappropriate activation of one or another element of the immune system. Hyperactivity is defined as either an immune response that is directed against targets to which the immune system is normally unreactive, or a prolonged and damaging inflammatory reaction generated against 'genuine' antigens. We start with the evidence for a genetic contribution to some hyperactivity disorders.

10.5 Genetic contribution to immune hyperactivity disorders

Genetically related **immune hyperactivity** is less clear-cut than congenital immune deficiency. A genetic contribution has been inferred from the statistical association of a number of mainly autoimmune diseases with the occurrence of particular alleles at certain *MHC* gene loci. The mechanisms by which the existence of a particular allele gives rise to the disease state is poorly understood for most of these conditions. We don't know why some people who have the 'increased risk' allele for a particular disorder remain well while others become ill, nor what triggers the onset of the condition, although environmental factors seem to be important.

You will recall from Figure 4.18 that the *MHC* genes in humans are termed the *HLA complex* and that the six major loci are *HLA-A, HLA-B, HLA-C*, and *HLA-DP, DQ* and *DR*. The great majority of *HLA*-associated diseases that have been identified are more common in individuals with particular alleles at the *HLA-DR* locus, as Table 10.1 shows.

TABLE 10.1 Association of *HLA* alleles with the occurrence of certain diseases in humans

Disease	*HLA* allele*	Relative risk**
dermatitis herpetiformis (an autoimmune skin disease)	DR3	56.4
insulin-dependent diabetes (autoimmune)	DR3/4	14.3
chronic active hepatitis (an autoimmune liver disease)	DR3	13.9
Goodpasture's syndrome (an autoimmune disease affecting the lungs and kidneys)	DR2	13.1
coeliac disease (involves hypersensitivity to gluten in wheat products)	DR3	10.8
Sjögren's syndrome (autoimmune destruction of salivary glands and tear ducts)	DR3	9.7
tuberculoid leprosy	DR2	8.1
Addison's disease (autoimmune destruction of adrenal cortex)	DR3	6.3
rheumatoid arthritis (autoimmune)	DR4	5.8
multiple sclerosis	DR2	4.8
thyrotoxicosis (autoimmune over-activity of thyroid gland)	DR3	3.7
Hashimoto's disease (autoimmune inflammation of the thyroid gland)	DR5	3.2
ankylosing spondilitis (progressive spinal deformity)	B27	87.4
Reiter's disease (arthritis of lower spine)	B27	37.0
post-infection arthritis (following infection with *Salmonella*, *Shigella*, *Yersinia*, or *Neisseria gonorrhoea*)	B27	14.0–29.7
subacute thyroiditis	Bw35	13.7
myasthenia gravis (autoimmune destruction of muscle receptors for neurotransmitters)	B8	4.4
psoriasis (a skin disease)	Cw6	13.3
haemochromatosis (excessive absorption of iron causing severe tissue damage)	A3	8.2

* Different *HLA* alleles are distinguished by a letter-and-number code. The first letter of the code denotes in which of the six major loci that allele occurs (e.g. *DR3* is an allele found in the *HLA-DR* locus).
** Relative risk indicates the increased chance of a person with this allele developing the disease compared to individuals with some other allele at this locus.

☐ Which molecules are coded for by *HLA-DR* and how could they be associated with susceptibility to disease?

■ *HLA-D* codes for the class II MHC molecules, which are involved in immune recognition of antigen by helper T cells. This region is homologous with the *I region* of the mouse *MHC*, and it is therefore thought to play a major role in regulating immune responsiveness. The diseases associated with particular alleles of the *HLA-D* region are primarily autoimmune conditions (Table 10.1), so the implication is that class II molecules are associating with self-epitopes in the cell membrane and somehow facilitating the activation of immune cells by epitopes that normally are tolerated.

Alleles at other *HLA* loci may also express surface molecules that associate with self-epitopes and generate 'foreign' conformations. Table 10.1 shows that several types of arthritic disease are associated with a particular allele at the *HLA-B* locus

(*B27*). One of these is a progressive deformity of the spine known as *ankylosing spondylitis*, which is virtually confined to people with the *B27* allele, but the mechanisms by which this gene causes the disorder remain a mystery. Other arthritic inflammatory disorders are mediated in part by the trapping of immune complexes in joints—a subject to which we turn in Section 10.6.

The association of hyperactivity disorders with certain genes *outside* the *HLA complex* has also been demonstrated, although less is understood about these conditions. For example, several of the autoimmune conditions listed in Table 10.1 are more likely to occur in members of the same family than in the general population, regardless of which *HLA* allele the family members have in the *D* region; this suggests that there is a genetic contribution to these conditions from outside the *HLA complex*. Two of the best described non-*HLA* associated congenital hyperactivity disorders produce defects in the proteases that break down complement components. They result either in widespread complement-mediated lysis of red blood cells (anaemia), or in fluid leaking from blood vessels into the tissues (oedema) as a result of the persistent action of complement.

10.6 Hypersensitivity reactions

Hypersensitivity reactions involve mechanisms that occur during the normal protective immune response to pathogens and parasites; but in certain individuals *either* the regulation processes break down *or* the antigen persists in the body. Under these circumstances, the immune response becomes exaggerated or pro-longed enough to cause significant tissue damage and unpleasant symptoms. Four types of hypersensitivity reaction have been classified according to their mechanisms, and hence according to which elements of the immune system are responding to antigen in an excessive or inappropriate manner. Types I, II and III are initiated by antibodies but type IV is initiated by helper T cells. However, more than one type can be found in the same individual at the same time, and this is generally the case with many autoimmune diseases. We will discuss autoimmune diseases in more detail at the end of this Chapter, but as you read the accounts of hypersensitivity reactions below consider the consequences if the antigen is a self-epitope.

10.6.1 Type I: immediate hypersensitivity

In Chapters 2 and 3 we described the inflammatory reaction triggered by IgE-mediated degranulation of mast cells, which is such an important part of the immune response to parasites. However, as we mentioned earlier, it also underlies the hay fever-like allergic response that is experienced by at least ten per cent of the population to normally harmless antigens such as pollens, house dust, animal fur and certain foods.

Type I hypersensitivity has a very rapid onset when the sensitised person is exposed to the allergen for a second or subsequent time, but no symptoms occur during the first exposure. When the allergen is encountered for the first time, IgE with binding sites for the allergen is secreted by particular clones of B cells. Free IgE becomes bound to mast cells via Fc-receptors on the surface membranes. The IgE remains attached to the mast cells until the second or subsequent exposure to the allergen, which is then able to cross-link adjacent molecules of IgE (Figure 10.2). This event triggers immediate mast cell degranulation, with the consequent oedema, redness, swelling and pain that characterise the acute inflammatory reaction (Figure 10.3).

Mast cells are particularly abundant in the respiratory tract and to a lesser extent in the walls of the gut, so it should come as no surprise to note that most allergens are either airborne or occur in food, and that type I hypersensitivity reactions are

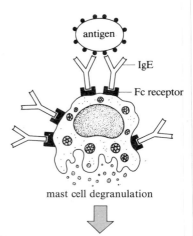

mast cell degranulation

acute inflammatory reaction

FIGURE 10.2 Immediate hypersensitivity (type I) triggered when IgE molecules linked to mast cells bind to their complementary antigen, causing mast cell degranulation and a local inflammatory reaction. The mechanism is part of the protective response to parasites, but can be triggered by otherwise innocuous antigens in sensitised people.

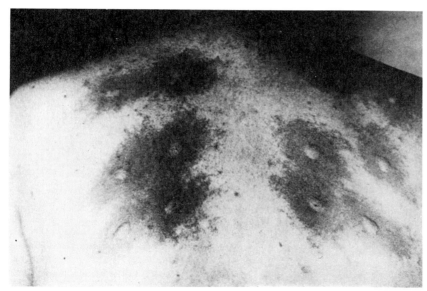

FIGURE 10.3 Immediate hypersensitivity response following injections of an allergen into the skin of a sensitised individual. A hot, red, tender swelling resembling a nettle sting developes within minutes around the injection sites.

usually confined to the respiratory tract and the gut. Airborne allergens typically produce constriction of the airways (bronchospasm). However, certain individuals may develop an allergy to a *systemic* antigen, that is, one that is disseminated throughout the body in the bloodstream. Penicillin and wasp or bee venom are the most common examples. Contact with such an antigen can prove very rapidly fatal to a sensitised individual because the chemicals released by mast cells produce a sudden dilation of blood capillaries (vasodilation), coupled with bronchospasm.

☐   Why could this reaction prove fatal?

■   Widespread vasodilation causes a sudden drop in blood pressure and reduces the supply of oxygen to the brain; bronchospasm produces an intense constriction of the airways, and death is most commonly from asphyxiation. (An injection of adrenalin causes vasoconstriction and bronchodilation, and reverses the process if administered swiftly enough.)

There may be a genetic component in the development of allergies because the incidence is greater in people with close relatives who are allergy sufferers. This may be mediated via deregulation of genes coding for IgE, since the level of IgE in the serum is the best indicator of whether a person is likely to develop an allergy. However, the relationship between IgE levels and allergy is not straightforward; some allergy sufferers have normal IgE levels and many people with raised IgE never develop an allergy.

10.6.2   Type II: antibody-dependent cytotoxic hypersensitivity

In Chapters 2 and 3 of this Book we noted the role of IgG and IgM in making a bridge between target cells and the cytotoxic cells of the innate immune system (eosinophils and large granular lymphocytes). This enables the cytotoxic cells to kill infected host cells, as well as pathogens and parasites that would otherwise be resistant to them. The process is called *antibody-dependent cell-mediated cytotoxicity*, or ADCC for short. It also occurs when phagocytic cells (macrophages and neutrophils) bind via an antibody bridge to a target that is too large to engulf; this stimulates the phagocyte to empty its lysosomes on to the surface of the target cell. The third factor in ADCC is that IgG and IgM bound to target cells trigger the complement cascade, with all its consequent chemotactic and inflammatory effects.

Figure 10.4 summarises the elements of ADCC, but the reason for restating the features of this protective response here is that certain antigens provoke an intense and prolonged ADCC hypersensitivity, mediated by IgG or IgM and complement. The most common antigens to provoke type II hypersensitivity are human MHC molecules on the cells of transplants, and blood group antigens on transfused red cells. But several autoimmune diseases are also mediated principally by autoantibodies binding to self-epitopes and triggering an ADCC-type hypersensitivity reaction. Autoantibodies and complement are involved in the immune destruction of red blood cells (seen in haemolytic anaemia), in damage to the basement membranes of kidney glomeruli and the lung (Goodpasture's syndrome; Plate 10.1), and to the acetylcholine receptors on muscle end-plates (myasthenia gravis).

10.6.3 Type III: immune complex-mediated hypersensitivity

Complexes of antigen bound together by antibodies are normally eliminated by phagocytic cells. However, in certain circumstances the rate of immune-complex formation can be so great that it exceeds the rate of elimination, and complexes become trapped in the fine capillary beds of the kidneys (see Plate 10.2) and lungs, as well as in joints and in the skin. This sets off an inflammatory reaction mediated by complement and phagocytic cells (Figure 10.5). Type III hypersensitivity reactions are very commonly found in many autoimmune diseases, in which immune complexes consisting of self-epitopes and autoantibodies may be generated in large amounts.

Immune complexes are also involved in hypersensitivity reactions to chronic infection by persistent foreign antigens, for example, malarial parasites (*Plasmodium* species), *Mycobacterium leprae* or *Trypanosoma* species. Persistent inhalation of antigens can also cause type III hypersensitivity, as in Farmer's lung disease and Pigeon Fancier's disease, so called because immune complexes form to antigens in mouldy hay or pigeon droppings respectively.

☐   Before antibiotics and vaccines were available to treat commonly fatal infections such as diphtheria, large quantities of antibodies to these pathogens were raised mainly in horses, and the antisera were injected into patients. What would be the result of this?

■   Initially the horse antibodies would form immune complexes with the antigen to which they were directed, but subsequently they would themselves become the target for antibodies raised in the patient against horse immunoglobulins. This would result in large amounts of immune complexes being deposited in the kidneys and other capillary beds. (The type III hypersensitivity that ensued was known as *serum sickness*.)

10.6.4 Type IV: delayed or cell-mediated hypersensitivity

Unlike types I to III, type IV hypersensitivity is mediated initially by T cells and subsequently by other effector cells attracted to the site of the reaction by lymphokines (Figure 10.6). As with all the hypersensitivity reactions, type IV is an exaggerated version of a protective cell-mediated immune response. The T cells are members of the helper subset that have become sensitised to the antigen at a previous encounter. Some texts classify them as a separate subset—the **delayed hypersensitivity T cells**.

Type IV hypersensitivity reactions take days or weeks to develop in sensitised individuals, in contrast with types I to III, which have a more rapid onset (hence the alternative term, *delayed* hypersensitivity, for type IV). Two broad groups of type IV reactions can be distinguished in previously sensitised individuals. The first

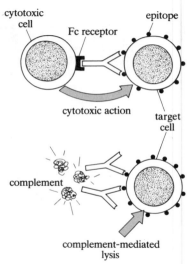

FIGURE 10.4 Antibody-dependent cytotoxic hypersensitivity (type II), mediated by cytotoxic cells, IgG or IgM and complement. The mechanism is the same as antibody-dependent cell-mediated cytotoxicity (ADCC), but is either prolonged and damaging to normal tissues in the region of the target cells, or is directed against inappropriate targets, such as the body's own cells.

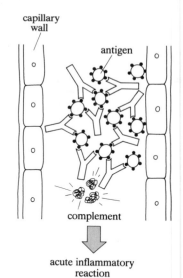

FIGURE 10.5 Immune complex-mediated hypersensitivity (type III). When immune complexes are formed in very large amounts they become lodged in capillaries and joints and trigger the complement cascade and a local inflammatory reaction. This type of hypersensitivity arises most commonly when large amounts of soluble antigen are continuously presented to the immune system. Self-antigens often elicit this type of reaction.

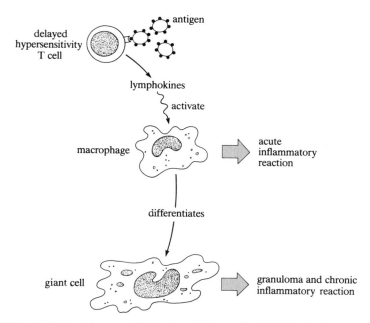

FIGURE 10.6 Delayed hypersensitivity (type IV) is mediated by T cells from the helper subset, which activate macrophages and trigger a delayed acute inflammatory reaction in response to certain skin-contact or bacterial antigens. Prolonged exposure to localised antigens (e.g. those on a parasite) can cause chronic (persistent) inflammation and granuloma formation by giant cells.

consists of *contact hypersensitivity* and *tuberculin hypersensitivity*, which develop within two to three days to an antigen applied to or injected into the skin of a sensitised individual. The second, *granulomatous hypersensitivity*, develops in response to persistent infection and may not be detectable for several weeks.

Contact hypersensitivity describes the intense local inflammatory skin reaction to antigens such as nickel, chemicals found in rubber or used in leather tanning, or poison ivy. The reaction is localised to the exact area that was in contact with the antigen (Figure 10.7). *Tuberculin* hypersensitivity develops in response to the injection of an antigen derived from *M. tuberculosis*. This is the basis of the Mantoux test given to schoolchildren in the UK to see if they are already sensitised by prior exposure to the bacterium (failure to develop a hypersensitivity reaction to the antigen implies no previous exposure and necessitates vaccination against tuberculosis). A similar type of reaction can be provoked by injecting antigen from other infectious organisms such as *M. leprae* into immune or infected individuals.

Granulomatous hypersensitivity is a much more serious disorder than the faster, generally self-limiting, delayed reactions to skin contact or antigens injected into the skin. It occurs when macrophages become persistently infected with intracellular pathogens or protozoa that they cannot eliminate. Lymphokines synthesised by neighbouring T cells stimulate the macrophages to undergo further differentiation into *giant* (or *epithelioid*) *cells*, and these aggregate into densely packed tissue swellings known as *granulomas*, which 'wall off' the infection in an area of intense inflammation. If the pathogens are successfully destroyed by this reaction the granuloma subsides, but if the infection persists then the granuloma becomes chronic and very serious tissue damage can result (Figure 10.8). Persistent infection with the pathogens that cause leprosy or tuberculosis, or with the leishmania or schistosome parasites commonly provokes a delayed granulomatous hypersensitivity reaction, which can result in severe tissue destruction.

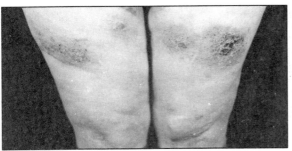

(a)

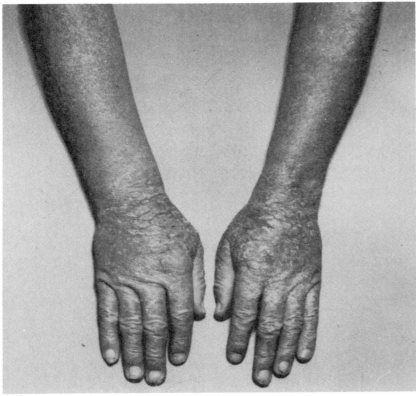

(b)

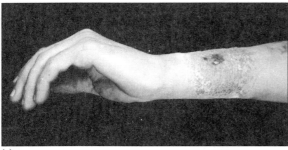

(c)

FIGURE 10.7 Contact hypersensitivity (delayed, cell-mediated, type IV) in the skin of people sensitive to (a) the nickel in suspender clips; (b) chemicals in adhesive resin; and (c) chemicals in a leather watch strap.

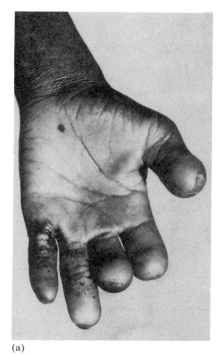
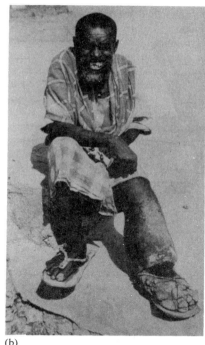

(a)   (b)

FIGURE 10.8 Chronic delayed hypersensitivity reactions contribute to the tissue damage seen in (a) the hand of a person infected with *M. leprae*, the causative agent of leprosy; and (b) the leg of a person infected with one of several species of filarial worm (the disease filariasis used to be known as 'elephantiasis', for obvious reasons). In both cases, the tissue damage results from chronic granulomas which form around the site of infection, preventing it from spreading but also cutting off the blood supply to that region.

10.7 Autoimmune diseases

We conclude this Chapter, and this Book, with a few statements summarising the many points that we have already made in relation to **autoimmune diseases**. We have discussed at some length the mechanisms by which the immune system develops tolerance to self, and summarised current theories about the reasons underlying the breakdown of self-tolerance (Chapter 8). The involvement of the *HLA complex* and other unidentified genes in the activation of self-reactive B cells or T cells has been suggested above, and we can add that the incidence of autoimmune disease rises with age, which may indicate that accumulated mutations might also play a part. The damage inflicted on cells and tissues in an autoimmune disease is very largely due to hypersensitivity reactions involving self-epitopes and autoantibodies or self-reactive T cells, as described in Section 10.6.

Autoimmune diseases can be grouped broadly into those that affect a single organ or tissue, and those that have widespread effects throughout the body. The damage in organ-specific autoimmune diseases is caused by autoantibodies or cytotoxic cells directed against epitopes found only on the cells of that organ (*tissue-specific antigens* were mentioned in Chapter 6). The thyroid gland, adrenal glands, pancreas, lungs, kidneys, salivary glands and stomach can all be affected by one or more organ-specific autoimmune diseases, some of which were listed in Table 10.1. Not mentioned in Table 10.1. (because it shows no association with particular HLA alleles) is *pernicious anaemia* resulting from autoantibodies that bind to and neutralise *intrinsic factor* in the gut. Intrinsic factor is essential for vitamin B_{12} absorption from the diet and hence for red blood cell development. Organ-specific autoimmunity has been found to underlie some cases of male infertility which are due to autoantibodies to spermatozoa, and premature menopause in some women is caused by autoantibodies to the cells that secrete *follicle stimulating hormone*.

It is important to note that although the majority of autoimmune states result in a *reduction* in the normal output or function of the affected organ, a few result in inappropriate *stimulation* of normal physiological mechanisms. The best described is autoimmune *thyrotoxicosis*, in which autoantibodies bind to receptors for thyroid stimulating hormone (TSH) on thyroid cells. This mimics the action of TSH and the result is hyperactivity of the thyroid gland, with all the consequent enhancement of metabolic processes. By contrast, *Hashimoto's thyroiditis* is caused by autoantibodies directed against thyroglobulin (from which the thyroid hormones are derived), which leads to an inflammatory reaction, the infiltration of the thyroid gland by huge numbers of immune cells, and severe damage to the gland.

Non-organ specific autoimmune diseases involve antibodies directed against epitopes found on cells throughout the body. Perhaps the most striking example is *systemic lupus erythematosus (SLE)*, in which autoantibodies from several B cell clones bind to epitopes on DNA, RNA and nuclear proteins. The symptoms are extremely varied and include inflammation of the skin and articular joints, and kidney disease, both caused by the trapping of large amounts of immune complexes in capillary beds in these locations. Patients with SLE often develop a characteristic facial skin rash due to inflammation triggered by immune complexes (Figure 10.9). This rash was thought to resemble the facial markings of the wolf—hence the inclusion of the Latin word *lupus*, meaning 'wolf', in the name given to this condition.

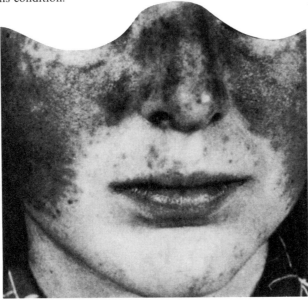

FIGURE 10.9 Characteristic facial skin inflammation caused by autoantibodies and immune complex-mediated hypersensitivity in a person with systemic lupus erythematosus (SLE).

Rheumatoid arthritis is another systemic autoimmune disease. It is characterised by the unrestrained growth of the synovial cells lining the joints, which is provoked by an intense immune response that includes the production of large amounts of antibody and immune complexes (Figure 10.10).

In conclusion, it must be stressed that we are still a very long way away from understanding what triggers an autoimmune disease, why affected people often have more than one such condition simultaneously, and why the symptoms classically wax and wane. A better understanding of the underlying mechanisms is essential to developing treatment strategies for controlling these often intractable and distressing conditions. Autoimmune diseases represent one of many stimuli from medical, academic and commercial sources for further research into the cells and molecules of the immune system.

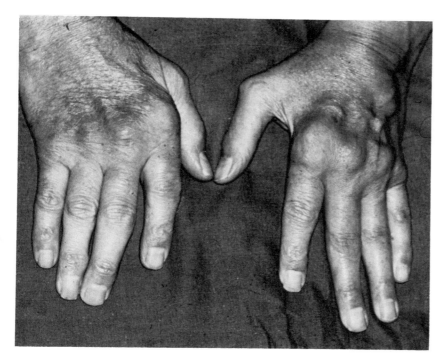

FIGURE 10.10 Rheumatoid arthritis affecting joints in the hands. Autoantibodies and immune complexes trigger chronic inflammation and excessive growth of synovial cells in the joints in this severely disabling and painful condition.

Summary of Chapter 10

1 Immune disorders may result from either a deficiency or a hyperactivity of the immune response. Some types of immunopathology have a genetic basis or contribution, whereas others are provoked by external agents.

2 Immune deficiencies may be congenital; or artificially induced by radiation or drugs used to prevent rejection of transplants or to treat cancers; or they may be induced by parasites or the human immunodeficiency virus (HIV). Immune deficiency leaves the person vulnerable to opportunistic infections.

3 Cancer cells do not, in general, proliferate as a result of immune deficiency. Malignant cells express oncogenes that were appropriately expressed in embryonic cells, and so cancer cells regain the ability to proliferate and migrate around the body. In the future, monoclonal antibodies may be targeted therapeutically on to onco-foetal antigens.

4 Many disorders of immune hyperactivity, especially autoimmune and arthritic diseases mediated by immune complexes, are associated with certain *HLA* alleles and/or kinship, but the mechanisms underlying the genetic contribution to these disorders are poorly understood.

5 Four types of hypersensitivity reaction have been classified, all of which are prolonged or inappropriately-targeted expressions of normal immune responses. Type I involves IgE-mediated mast cell degranulation in response to common environmental allergens. Type II involves antibody-dependent cell-mediated cytotoxicity to self-epitopes or to grafts and transfusions. Type III involves immune complexes arising from autoimmunity or persistent exposure to certain microbial or environmental antigens. And type IV involves T cell-mediated inflammatory reactions to antigens in the skin, or chronic granuloma formation in reaction to chronic infection.

6 Autoimmune diseases have a wide spectrum of symptoms, but most commonly involve some degree of hypersensitivity mediated by self-epitopes and autoantibodies or self-reactive T cells. The self-epitopes, and hence the tissue damage, may be confined to certain organs or they may be more widely distributed in the body.

Now attempt SAQs 36–38, which relate to this Chapter.

SELF-ASSESSMENT QUESTIONS (SAQs)

Chapter 1

SAQ 1

(a) Suppose that a strain of pathogen (strain A) was introduced into a tank containing an annelid worm, which became infected with strain A for a time but on examination several weeks later was found to be free from infection. What types of cell would be involved in eliminating the infection?

(b) Suppose that some time later the same worm became infected again with pathogens of strain A and *also* with pathogens of a closely related strain B. What differences (if any) would you expect in the response of the worm to these two strains, and why?

SAQ 2

Explain why infectious diseases that are common among British children (such as chickenpox and measles, both of which are caused by virus infections) are generally not suffered twice by the same person. Would you expect a person who has recovered from measles to be less susceptible to infection with chickenpox than a person who has never suffered from measles? Explain your answer.

SAQ 3

What situations, other than the immune deficiency state caused by HIV (the virus that can lead to AIDS), leave a person vulnerable to pathogens that would normally be eliminated by the immune response?

Chapter 2

SAQ 4

The serum of guinea pigs contains a high concentration of complement and is often used as a source of complement in laboratory experiments. If guinea pig serum were added to a culture dish containing live unencapsulated bacteria, what do you predict might happen? What might be the effect of adding guinea pig macrophages to the culture dish at a later time? (You can assume that the culture conditions are appropriate for maintaining viable bacteria and macrophages.)

SAQ 5

What is a *chemotactic factor* and what are the main sources and types of chemotactic factor in higher vertebrates?

SAQ 6

Three babies are born, each with a (hypothetical) defect in white cell development. Baby A is left without *macrophages*, baby B without *eosinophils*, and baby C without *NK cells*. As they grow up, what types of infectious organism are most likely to cause problems to each of these babies, and which of them is likely to have the most serious health problems?

SAQ 7

What similarity exists between the role of *interferons* and the role of *NK cells* in innate immunity? Describe one similarity and one difference in their mode of action.

Chapter 3

SAQ 8

The Human Immunodeficiency Virus (HIV)—the virus that can lead to AIDS—infects cells with surface CD4 molecules. The HIV virus particle has surface receptors that bind to CD4 molecules. CD4-binding is an essential prerequisite for the entry of viral nucleic acid into the cell. Cells with surface CD4 are thus susceptible to destruction as the virus replicates. What effect would you expect this to have on the function of the adaptive and innate immune responses over time?

SAQ 9

In the disease known as *agammaglobulinaemia* the affected person cannot synthesise antibodies, usually because their B cells are defective. But a minority of people with this condition have normal B cells that nevertheless fail to make antibodies to the antigens that enter the body. Suggest two possible causes, in terms of defects in other cell types, for this minority condition.

SAQ 10

Figure Q1 represents three laboratory cultures: X, Y and Z. The cells in each of these cultures are from the same individual and therefore express the same MHC molecules at the cell surface. The cultures have been incubated under ideal conditions for several hours, and the cells have gradually settled to the bottom of the culture vessels so that it is easy to remove cell-free supernatants from the vessel with a pipette.

(a)   What will happen in culture X?

(b)   Could the cell-free supernatant from *either* culture Y *or* culture Z alone induce lysis of the virus-infected cells if added to culture X? Could these two supernatants *mixed together* induce lysis in culture X?

(c)   Is there any way to induce lysis in culture X by the transfer of cell-free supernatants between the culture vessels if neither of the strategies in (b) is successful?

In each case, explain your answer carefully.

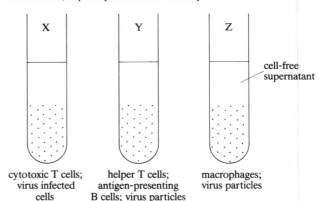

cytotoxic T cells;
virus infected
cells

helper T cells;
antigen-presenting
B cells; virus particles

macrophages;
virus particles

cell-free
supernatant

FIGURE Q1 Three different cell cultures: X, Y and Z. All the cells in the culture come from the same strain of mouse, and all the virus particles are from a single strain.

SAQ 11

Figure Q2 summarises an important experiment performed in 1974 by immunologists Ralph Zinkernagel and Peter Doherty. The two strains of mice differ in their class I MHC molecules because they have inherited different alleles of the genes in the *major histocompatibility complex*. Both strains were injected with virus Q and, some time later, virus-infected cells were removed and grown in cell cultures. Cytotoxic T cells from each strain, and the appropriate lymphokines necessary to activate them, were later added to the culture vessels in the combinations shown in the Figure. What outcome would you expect in each of the culture vessels and why?

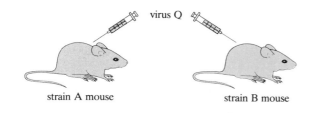

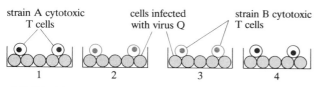

FIGURE Q2 Culture vessels 1 and 2 contain cells infected with virus Q from mouse strain A; culture vessels 3 and 4 contain cells infected with virus Q from mouse strain B. Culture vessels 1 and 4 also contain cytotoxic T cells from strain A, whereas vessels 2 and 3 contain cytotoxic T cells from strain B.

SAQ 12

The enzyme *papain* splits antibody molecules into three parts: two identical Fab regions and one Fc region per antibody molecule. Suppose that antibodies to *Streptococcus pneumoniae* (an encapsulated strain of bacteria that can cause pneumonia) were treated with papain and then added to a tissue culture containing these bacteria, together with macrophages and neutrophils.

(a) What outcome would you expect, and how would this compare with the outcome in a similar culture that contained intact antibodies to the bacteria?

(b) What would be the effect of adding guinea pig serum (which is rich in complement) to either of these cultures? Carefully explain your answers.

SAQ 13

Where in the body would you expect to find human T cells, B cells and macrophages (a) before and (b) after exposure to an appropriate antigen?

Chapter 4

SAQ 14

A colony of syngeneic mice were divided into two groups: A and B. Group A mice were injected with a hapten to which they had never previously been exposed, and group B mice were injected with the *same* hapten linked to a suitable carrier molecule. After 28 days both groups of mice were injected with the hapten–carrier conjugate, and every two days thereafter their serum was tested for the presence of antibodies that bind to epitopes on the hapten. What differences, if any, would you expect to find in the antibody response of each group of mice following this second injection? Give reasons for your answer.

SAQ 15

Rearrange the following events into the correct chronological sequence resulting in the synthesis of kappa (κ) light chains and their incorporation into an antibody molecule.

(a) A primary mRNA transcript is made of the *V* gene adjacent to the remaining *J* genes, together with the remaining *J* genes and the light-chain *C* gene.

(b) A pair of identical kappa light chains becomes covalently linked to a pair of identical heavy chains.

(c) The germ-line gene sets coding for lambda light chains are suppressed, together with either the maternal or paternal germ-line genes coding for kappa light chains.

(d) A mature mRNA transcript is translated into a kappa light chain with a unique variable region.

(e) Alternative *J* genes are excised by cutting and splicing, together with the non-coding and leader sequences transcribed from the recombined B cell DNA.

(f) Somatic recombination during differentiation of a mature B cell from the germ-line cell results in excision of the DNA intervening between a selected *V* gene and a selected *J* gene.

SAQ 16

Read the following statements and decide which (if any) are wholly or partly false. Formulate a correct statement for any that you judge to be incorrect.

(a) The valency of the normally occurring form of antibodies in each immunoglobulin class is two.

(b) Variable domains from IgG molecules obtained from the *same* B cell show a high degree of variability in their primary structure when one molecule is compared with another.

(c) Constant domains from immunoglobulin heavy chains show a high degree of similarity in their higher-order structure, and in parts of their primary structure, with particular domains in the MHC molecules and in the T cell antigen receptor.

(d) All five immunoglobulin classes can trigger the complement cascade, but only IgG molecules can pass across the placenta from mother to foetus.

(e) IgA is the principal antibody class found in secretions on mucous membranes lining the lungs and gut, and also in sweat, tears and saliva.

(f) Each B cell can either synthesise antibodies with two kappa light chains or with two lambda light chains, but hybrid antibody molecules with a kappa and a lambda light chain never occur in life.

(g) The recognition of 'self' MHC class II molecules in association with viral antigens leads to the destruction of virus-infected body cells by cytotoxic T cells.

(h) The principal molecular assemblies that can bind to antigen in a specific way are complexes of from three to at least five dissimilar transmembrane polypeptide chains held together by covalent bonds.

SAQ 17

Distinguish between *syngeneic* and *congenic* mice and deduce how congenic strains may be used to map the locations and functions of the major *MHC* loci.

SAQ 18

Would you expect antibodies, MHC molecules and T cell receptors involved in recognising a particular antigen to bind to the *same* epitope on that antigen? Explain your answer.

Chapter 5

SAQ 19

Figure Q3 illustrates the appearance of antibodies to influenza virus antigens in the bloodstream of mice infected with the virus. In what ways might adaptive and innate mechanisms contribute to the reduction in virus concentration *before* serum antibodies reach measurable levels?

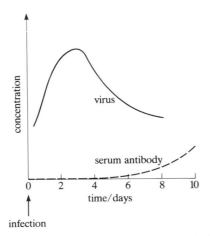

FIGURE Q3 Appearance of anti-viral antibodies in the serum of mice infected for the first time with influenza virus follows several days *after* a decline in virus concentration has occurred.

SAQ 20

Human babies born with an extremely rare condition known as *Di George syndrome* have no thymus gland. Which types of pathogen or parasite would you expect these babies to be particularly vulnerable to, and why?

SAQ 21

The virus that causes the common cold exists as hundreds of different strains, each with slightly different surface antigens. How does this contribute to the survival of the virus and what problems does it raise for vaccine development? What relationship would you predict between a person's *age* and the *incidence* of common colds (i.e. the number of colds that they suffer per year)? Explain your answer.

Chapter 6

SAQ 22

Under favourable conditions, soluble antigens can be precipitated from solution if enough antigen molecules are cross-linked by antibodies directed against their epitopes. Precipitation is therefore evidence of antigen–antibody binding. The following experiment with a hypothetical antigen makes use of this.

Antigen X is a globular protein that is soluble in water. Each molecule of antigen X has only two epitopes, which are structurally so different that antibodies with binding sites for epitope 1 will not bind to epitope 2, and vice versa. An antiserum containing a mixture of Ig-1 (which binds to epitope 1) and Ig-2 (which binds to epitope 2) was obtained by injecting antigen X into mice. Antigen X can be cleaved into fragments by enzymes. A peptide fragment containing a loop stabilised by a disulphide bond (the *loop* peptide) was split from antigen X, and this in turn can be freed from the loop conformation by reducing the disulphide bond (to give the *linear* peptide).

The antiserum raised against antigen X was tested for its ability to precipitate a solution of the *intact* antigen (experiment A below), the *loop* peptide (experiment B) and the *linear* peptide (experiment C). In experiments D and E the antiserum was tested for its ability to precipitate intact antigen X in the presence of an *excess* of either the loop peptide or the linear peptide. Study the results of each of these experiments in Table Q1 and then answer questions (a) to (e), which follow.

TABLE Q1 Experimental results

| | Test-tube contents: | | | |
Experiment	antiserum	intact antigen X	excess peptide	Precipitation
A	+	+	−	+
B	+	−	loop	−
C	+	−	linear	−
D	+	+	loop	−
E	+	+	linear	+

(a) The antiserum was able to precipitate intact antigen X (experiment A). Draw a rough sketch showing how the antibodies in the antiserum could cross-link the molecules of antigen X.

(b) Neither of the peptides *alone* was able to form a precipitate with the antiserum (experiments B and C). Give two possible reasons for this.

(c) How do the results of experiments D and E help to distinguish between the two alternative explanations that you outlined in (b) above?

(d) What reason can you give for the fact that excess *loop* peptide could inhibit precipitation of antigen X by the antiserum, but excess *linear* peptide could not? (experiments D and E).

(e) Explain why the loop peptide *on its own* could not form a precipitate with the antiserum (experiment B) but could *inhibit* the precipitation of the intact antigen if present in excess (experiment D).

SAQ 23

Hen egg-white lysozyme is a globular protein with several epitopes in its structure, which are immunogenic in mice. Table Q2 divides the amino acids found in some of these epitopes into three groups. What is the characteristic shared by the members of a group, and what conclusions can be drawn about epitopes from the data in the Table?

TABLE Q2 Amino acids involved in some of the epitopes in the structure of hen egg-white lysozyme

Group	Amino acids	Total number of residues
1	arginine, lysine, aspartic acid and glutamic acid	11
2	phenylalanine, tryptophan	2
3	asparagine, threonine	3

SAQ 24

Which of the combinations of donor and recipient given in Table Q3 would provoke a transfusion reaction if blood was transfused from the donor to the recipient, and why?

TABLE Q3   Blood transfusion combinations

Blood group of donor	Blood group of recipient
A	B
B	AB
O	A
AB	B
A	O

Chapter 7

SAQ 25

If you wanted to produce a polyclonal antiserum containing antibodies that bound to the Fc region of human IgG how would you go about it? Why is a polyclonal antiserum relatively straightforward to produce against this particular antigen?

SAQ 26

If a *large* volume of soluble diphtheria toxin (the antigen) is added slowly to a *constant* volume of antitoxin (the antibodies), what would you expect to happen as the antigen concentration rises and why? You should describe three distinct phases in your answer.

SAQ 27

Use the data in Table Q4 below to plot the standard curves obtained from a radial immunodiffusion assay (RID) in which serial dilutions of human IgG (the antigen) were allowed to diffuse into a gel containing a standard concentration of anti-human IgG antibodies. The diameter of the precipitin ring was measured for each antigen dilution after 16 hours and again after 48 hours. What conclusions can you draw from these standard curves?

TABLE Q4   Results of a RID assay of standard concentrations of human IgG

	Ring diameter squared, d^2/mm:	
Human IgG units	after 16 hours	after 48 hours
100	90	130
50	60	74
25	40	46
12.5	30	32

After plotting the graph, use it to calculate the concentration of IgG in a human serum that gives a d^2 reading of 68 mm in a RID assay.

SAQ 28

Compare *immunoelectrophoresis* with *immunoblotting* in terms of (a) the different molecular characteristics of antigens that are exploited in these methods of protein separation, and (b) the way in which the separated antigens are identified in each case.

SAQ 29

Explain how you would carry out an enzyme-linked immunosorbent assay (ELISA) for anti-rubella virus antibodies in a person's serum, using solid-phase antigens and an *indirect* labelling method. Draw a sketch to illustrate your answer. (This test is performed to discover if a person has immunity to rubella, which causes German measles.)

Chapter 8

SAQ 30

The colostrum produced by the mammary glands in the first few days after birth contains antibodies to many antigens that the mother has encountered during her life, and these antibodies are also found to a lesser extent in breast milk. What is the significance of this for the health of the new-born baby?

SAQ 31

Summarise two alternative models for the sequence of events in the thymus that culminates in the maturation of T cells restricted to recognise antigen only in association with self-MHC molecules (i.e. self-MHC restriction).

SAQ 32

Figure Q4 shows the results of an experiment to test the specificity of artificial tolerance induction. Three groups of syngeneic mice were used: A, B and C. On the first day of the experiment, group A were injected with an inert solution, group B were injected with 1.0 mg of a polysaccharide antigen known as B512, and group C were injected with 10.0 mg of B512. This antigen has a single epitope X in its structure. After 14 days, all three groups of mice were injected with a small immunogenic dose of another polysaccharide antigen, B1355, which also has epitope X and another epitope Y in its structure. On day 19, the number of plasma cells producing antibodies to either epitope X or to epitope Y in the spleen of animals in each group was estimated. Study Figure Q4 and interpret the results of the experiment.

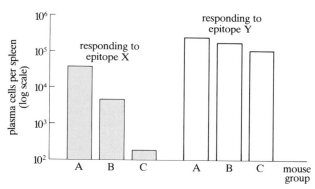

FIGURE Q4   Results of the experiment described in SAQ 32.

Chapter 9

SAQ 33

Distinguish between three functional subsets of helper T cells: the inducers of suppression, the inducers of help, and the contrasuppressors.

SAQ 34

Describe two ways in which circuits of immune cells could (in theory) achieve *antigen-specific* suppression of a particular clone of B cells.

SAQ 35

Figure Q5 gives the protocol for an experiment to investigate the phenomenon of self-MHC restriction in the cooperation between immune cells. Study the protocol carefully and then answer the following questions.

(a) Describe the lymphocytes that were removed from the *H-2^d* mouse after it had been irradiated, injected with *H-2^d* thymus cells, and then injected with antigen Q. Explain how you arrived at your answer.

(b) Describe the lymphocytes that were removed from the *H-2^k* mouse after they had been treated with anti-T cell antibodies and complement.

(c) Would you expect the lymphocytes that were injected into the *H-2$^{d/k}$* mouse to survive?

(d) What do you predict will happen when the reconstituted *H-2$^{d/k}$* mouse is challenged with antigen Q? Explain your answer carefully.

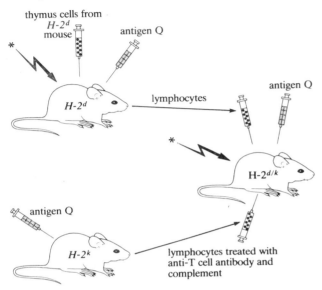

FIGURE Q5 Protocol for the experiment associated with SAQ 35. The irradiation symbols denote that the mice were X-irradiated to destroy all their immune cells *before* they were reconstituted with lymphocytes and injected with antigen Q.

Chapter 10

SAQ 36
Summarise the main problems in developing *vaccines* to protect people against HIV infection or *drugs* to treat existing HIV infection. (Note: you will have to think back to the earlier discussion of viral escape strategies in Chapter 5 for part of your answer.)

SAQ 37
Babies born to women who suffer from *autoimmune thyrotoxicosis* or *myasthenia gravis* show, respectively, a transient hyperactivity of the thyroid gland or a transient muscle weakness in the days following birth, before developing normal function. Explain these phenomena.

SAQ 38
All four types of hypersensitivity can be detected in the normal immune response to certain *parasites*. Explain the mechanisms involved.

ANSWERS TO SAQs

SAQ 1

(a) Phagocytic cells in the body of the worm could engulf the pathogens and destroy them, and cytotoxic cells could secrete toxic or membrane-puncturing chemicals on to the pathogens. Some form of primitive antibody molecule (antisome) may also be formed, which would bind to the pathogens, aiding their destruction by phagocytosis.

(b) The immune system of the worm would not adapt during the first immune response to strain A. Put another way, it would not retain an immunological memory of the structure of strain A, and so it would respond in exactly the same way with the same degree of effectiveness when it became infected with strain A for a second time. It cannot distinguish between strain A and strain B, since primitive immune cells have only general receptors for foreign material, so it will respond to both strains in exactly the same way. This form of immunity is known as *innate immunity*.

SAQ 2

Humans are higher vertebrates and therefore have adaptive immunity as well as innate immunity. When a child becomes infected for the first time, with (say) the virus that causes measles, cells in the adaptive immune system that have receptors of the correct shape bind to epitopes on the virus, and a *primary* adaptive response is directed specifically against the virus particles. After the virus has been eliminated, the immune system remains permanently adapted to mount a faster, more effective *secondary* response against the measles virus if the same epitopes are ever encountered again. Thus, it is unusual for someone to suffer twice from measles because he or she will become *immune* to the virus after the first exposure.

However, the immune system is *not* adapted to respond more effectively to any other pathogen because each pathogen has different epitopes and the immune system recognises each one specifically. So a person who has *recovered* from measles is just as likely to suffer from (say) chickenpox for the first time as a person who has never had measles. Protection against one infectious disease generally does not give protection against another, unless the epitopes on the two strains are very similar (as is the case with the smallpox and cowpox viruses—the first experiments with vaccination successfully used live cowpox virus to immunise a child against smallpox).

SAQ 3

The effectiveness of the immune system is undermined by malnutrition and multiple infections (as is often the case in Third World countries), so the person becomes susceptible to infections that he or she would be able to fight off if in good health. In transplantation medicine, the immune system may be artificially suppressed with drugs so that the patient's body accepts an organ graft from an unrelated person; this renders patients particularly susceptible to infection, so they are isolated in a clean environment while they recover.

SAQ 4

If the polysaccharide groups in the bacterial cell wall were of the type that activate the first component of complement, then the cascade reaction would be triggered. (Note that *unencapsulated* bacteria can generally activate complement whereas encapsulated bacteria cannot because their cell wall is concealed). The end-product of the complement cascade is the membrane attack complex, which punches holes in the bacterial cell wall. If enough pores were made then the bacteria would die, but it is likely that this would be a rather slow process. However, bacterial destruction could be greatly speeded up if macrophages were added to the culture. They bind readily to bacteria that have been *opsonised* by C3b (one of the components of the activated complement system), and then kill the bacteria by phagocytosis.

SAQ 5

Chemotactic factors attract white cells by acting as chemical 'beacons'. The white cells 'home in' on the source of the factor by migrating up the concentration gradient. In higher vertebrates, chemotactic factors are secreted mainly by macrophages and mast cells, or as components of the complement cascade (G5a is one of the most potent).

SAQ 6

Baby A would be in the most trouble because macrophages not only *phagocytose* bacteria, viruses, fungi and protozoa, but also manufacture and secrete *interferons*, some of the components of *complement*, *lysozyme*, *chemotactic factors* and factors involved in increasing the *permeability* of capillaries in the inflammatory reaction. Defects of macrophage development do exist and can prove fatal. Baby B might have more difficulty eliminating multicellular parasites than a normal baby, but the immune response to parasites is not very successful at best, so the difference might not be critical. Baby C might have more trouble eliminating virus infections than a normal baby, but NK cells form less than one per cent of white cells and there are many other mechanisms for dealing with virus infections, so again this might not be a critical defect.

SAQ 7

Interferons and NK cells have a similar *role* in innate immunity in that both inhibit viruses from spreading from infected body cells to nearby uninfected ones. Similarities in their *mode of action* are that both are effective against *any* type of virus (i.e. both are *non-specifically* active against viruses), and neither has any activity against 'free' virus particles, bacteria, fungi or parasites. However, there is a major difference in their activity: interferons bind to *uninfected* cells and greatly reduce mRNA transcription, rendering the cell incapable of manufacturing new virus particles, whereas NK cells kill *infected* cells by perforating the target cell membrane and destroying an existing 'factory' of virus particles.

SAQ 8

CD4 molecules are the characteristic surface *marker* molecules on *helper* T cells, so HIV infection leads to the selective destruction of the helper subset. This has profound consequences for adaptive and innate immunity, both of which decline in effectiveness over time, because the lymphokines secreted by helper T cells (see Table 3.2) are essential for the activation, differentiation and proliferation of white cells involved in all aspects of an immune response. In the absence of helper T cells, innate immunity could (in theory) still proceed, but at a reduced intensity and effectiveness. Adaptive immunity against T cell-*dependent* antigens grinds to a halt, although T cell-independent antigens could still elicit a B cell response. (In fact, macrophages are one of the other cell types that HIV can infect, so the situation is even worse than predicted here; AIDS is discussed further in Chapter 10.)

SAQ 9

The two most obvious causes are (a) the absence or ineffectiveness of helper T cells, whose lymphokines are essential for the activation of most B cells; and (b) the over-activity of suppressor T cells, whose effect would be to inhibit B cells. You might also have considered a defect in antigen-presenting cells, which would lead to failure of helper T cell activation, with the same consequences as in (a). All three of these defects have been found in people with minority-type agammaglobulinaemia.

SAQ 10

(a) Cytotoxic T cells can only respond to the virus-infected cells in culture X if they receive activating signals in the form of various lymphokines secreted by helper T cells. Thus, nothing will happen in culture X.

(b) Culture Y contains helper T cells and antigen, but the supernatant does not contain the essential lymphokines because helper T cells won't secrete lymphokines unless they are stimulated by interleukin-1 (Il-1), which is secreted by macrophages. The supernatant from culture Z won't induce lysis in culture X because, although it *does* contain Il-1 secreted by the macrophages, it doesn't contain lymphokines (there are no helper T cells in culture Z). Mixing these two supernatants together makes no difference —this just transfers Il-1 on to cytotoxic T cells.

(c) The way round this is to *first* transfer supernatant from culture Z to culture Y and wait until the Il-1 from culture Z has activated the helper T cells in culture Y to start secreting lymphokines. *Then* the transfer of supernatant from culture Y to culture X should induce lysis of the virus-infected cells in culture X.

SAQ 11

Lysis of the virus-infected cells would occur only in vessels 1 and 3, which contain infected cells and cytotoxic T cells from the *same* mouse strain. Lysis would not occur in vessels 2 and 4 because the target cells and the cytotoxic T cells have different class I MHC molecules in their surface membrane. The cytotoxic T cells in vessels 2 and 4 cannot bind to the viral antigens because they are not presented in association with *self-MHC* molecules. The T cell receptor for antigen *simultaneously* binds to the epitope and to MHC molecules that are identical to those on the T cell itself. This was the first experiment to demonstrate the phenomenon of self-MHC restriction of T cells; it caused enormous excitement when it was published because the phenomenon was quite unexpected.

SAQ 12

(a) Papain treatment splits the antibody molecules into Fab regions, which bind to epitopes on the bacterial capsule, and Fc regions, which bind to the Fc receptors on the phagocytes. However, the split antibody molecules cannot act as *opsonins* because they cannot form a 'bridge' between the bacteria and the phagocytes. Phagocytosis would be very slow because encapsulated bacteria are difficult for macrophages and neutrophils to adhere to. In the culture with intact antibodies, the bacteria *are* opsonised, so phagocytosis would destroy them much more quickly.

(b) Adding complement to the culture with papain-treated antibodies would speed up the destruction of the bacteria *provided* that *Streptococcus pneumoniae* capsules contain the correct polysaccharide groups to trigger the complement cascade (Chapter 2). If so, then phagocytes may be attracted to the bacteria by C5a, the bacteria may be opsonised by C3b, or

perforated by the membrane attack complex. In the culture containing intact antibodies, the complement cascade *will* be activated powerfully by antibodies bound to the bacteria, all the possible outcomes described above will occur, and it will take much less time to destroy all the bacteria.

SAQ 13

(a) Before exposure to antigen you would expect to find memory T cells and B cells, naive T cells and at least some macrophages circulating in the lymphatic and vascular systems, and migrating through the tissues; the majority of the macrophages would be in the tissues, migrating back and forth to nearby lymph nodes, and the naive B cells would be stationary in the lymphoid organs.

(b) After exposure to antigen you would expect to find all these leukocytes attracted to the site of infection or to lymphoid organs in which antigen has been trapped. Macrophages are found contributing to inflammatory reactions in the tissues and 'presenting' antigen to T cells in the lymph nodes. Activated T and B cells migrate to the nearest peripheral lymphoid organ and remain there while an immune response is generated. A large proportion of B cells also migrate back into the bone marrow and become antibody-secreting *plasma cells* there.

SAQ 14

The main differences in the response of the two groups of mice to the second injection are that after about ten days, group A mice will produce mainly IgM antibodies with relatively low affinity for the hapten, whereas group B mice will produce a much higher concentration of mainly IgG antibodies within about three days and with much greater affinity for the hapten.

The explanation is as follows. The hapten alone is not immunogenic, so the mice in group A will not mount an immune response to the first injection. However, a primary immune response occurs in the mice in group B after exposure to the hapten–carrier conjugate, which *is* immunogenic. A primary response takes about 28 days to subside (Chapter 3), during which time the group B mice will form memory cells with surface bound IgM as receptors for the hapten. The *VDJ* immunoglobulin genes in the memory cell DNA are prone to somatic mutation during memory cell formation, so a range of receptors arises with greater or lesser affinity for the hapten. When the second injection of hapten–carrier conjugate is given to the group B mice, the hapten will bind preferentially to those memory cells that have receptors with the highest affinity. This ensures that the antibody-secreting plasma cells that proliferate from the selected memory cells synthesise antibodies with a higher affinity than those secreted during the primary response.

During the differentiation and proliferation of the secondary plasma cells in the group B mice, class switching takes place as a result of the cutting and splicing of the heavy-chain *C* genes (or their mRNA transcripts) to remove the genes coding for antibodies with IgM or IgD heavy chains. This recombination brings the gene coding for IgG heavy chains next to the *VDJ* genes, so the class of antibody secreted by these cells is IgG.

The second injection of the hapten (this time with a carrier) into the group A mice is responded to as though it were the first exposure; thus, a primary antibody response ensues, characterised by the slow production of relatively low affinity IgM.

SAQ 15

The correct chronological sequence is (c), (f), (a), (e), (d) and (b). Figure 4.13 shows the central parts of this sequence.

SAQ 16

Statements (c), (e) and (f) are true.

(a) is false because the valency of the normally occurring dimeric form of IgA is four, and of the pentameric form of IgM is ten.

(b) is false in that all the molecules of antibody made by the *same* B cell are identical; the statement would be correct only if it referred to *different* B cells.

(d) is false because only IgG and IgM trigger the complement cascade, but it correctly refers to IgG as the only class that can cross the placenta.

(g) refers to the wrong class of MHC molecule: class I molecules are involved in recognition by cytotoxic T cells.

(h) contains *four* errors. First, the number of different polypeptides in these molecular assemblies ranges from *two* to five or more: antibodies have four; MHC molecules have two; and the T cell receptor has five or more (TcR + CD3). Second, the chains are not all *dissimilar*: the light chains in the antibody molecule are identical, as are the heavy chains. Third, the polypeptide chains are held together by covalent bonds only in the case of the antibody molecule and the TcR dimer of the T cell receptor; all the other polypeptide chains are held together by non-covalent bonds. Fourth, not all of the chains in these polypeptides traverse the cell membrane: those that do *not* are the light chains of surface immunoglobulin and all four chains of secreted antibodies, and the β-chain of MHC class I molecules (i.e. β_2-microglobulin).

SAQ 17

Syngeneic mice are identical in all the alleles at every locus of the *MHC* genes; mice are described as *congenic* when they differ in the allele present at just *one MHC* locus. Congenic strains have been used in many kinds of investigation. For example, transplantation of tissue between congenic strains that differ at a known locus can identify which loci code for MHC molecules with epitopes that are the target for graft rejection. *In vitro* studies of the ability of cytotoxic T cells from one strain of mouse to kill virus-infected cells of a congenic strain can help to identify which *MHC* loci code for class I MHC molecules.

SAQ 18

Unless the antigen is a polymer that has repeating identical epitopes (for example, some bacterial polysaccharides; see Chapter 3), then these three molecular assemblies must bind to *different* epitopes on the antigen. There are two reasons for concluding this. First, there is little homology between the amino acid sequence of the variable domains of antibody molecules, MHC molecules and T cell receptors (only certain of the constant domains resemble each other in primary as well as higher-order structure); it follows that they must have different binding sites and hence must bind to different epitopes. Second, the T cell receptor and the MHC molecules bind to antigen *simultaneously*; therefore they cannot be binding to the same epitope.

SAQ 19

Figure Q6 shows the most important part of the answer.

Interferon produced by macrophages and helper T cells renders cells in the respiratory tract resistant to infection by the virus, so replication declines for want of suitable host cells. This is a collaborative venture because interferons also *activate* helper T cells, and T cells produce lymphokines, which *increase* the activity of macrophages. In addition, lung macrophages phagocytose a proportion of free virus particles, and cytotoxic T cells kill lung cells that are already infected. The mucosal surfaces of the lungs are also protected by IgA, so even though antibodies in the *serum* take several days to reach an appreciable level, the *local* concentration of IgA antibodies may be sufficient to contribute to the reduction in virus concentration.

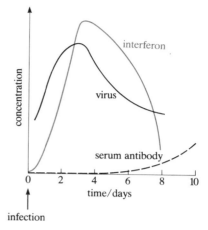

FIGURE Q6 The decline in virus concentration coincides with the appearance of high concentrations of interferon in the serum.

SAQ 20

The outlook is very poor for babies with Di George syndrome, who tend to succumb quite quickly to a wide range of infections. However, they show slightly more resistance to bacterial infections (especially those caused by Gram-positive bacteria) than they do to virus infections. The lack of a thymus means that they have no functional T cells, and this in turn leads to non-activation of most B cells in contact with antigens. Even though innate immunity operates far less effectively in the absence of lymphokines and antibodies, a response against some types of bacteria can be mounted by phagocytes, and this is more effective if the bacterium is not shielded by a capsule or if polysaccharides in the bacterial cell wall trigger the complement cascade. By contrast, the defence against intracellular viruses is reduced to the action of interferons secreted by macrophages, and the action of NK cells (there are no cytotoxic T cells), without the enhancing action of antibodies and lymphokines.

SAQ 21

The existence of many strains with slightly different antigens produces a similar effect to antigenic drift. This is because an individual who has recovered from an infection with one strain (and who therefore has adaptive immunity to it) will have little or no protection against a strain with different surface antigens. And as long as someone within sneezing range of an infected person is also susceptible to that strain, then the virus is ensured of survival. An effective vaccine would have to contain the antigens of all the different strains. As time goes on, each individual will encounter more and more of the various strains and so will be less and less likely to meet a new one. This explains why children suffer from the common cold more frequently than do young adults, and colds are even less common in elderly people who are otherwise in good health. However, the most immune individuals are also the oldest; as they die from other causes they are replaced with new-borns who 'top up' the pool with individuals who are susceptible to *all* the many strains of the common cold virus.

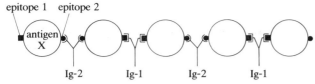

epitope 1   epitope 2

antigen
X

Ig-2   Ig-1   Ig-2   Ig-1

FIGURE Q7 Cross-linking of the divalent antigen X by two species of antibodies, Ig-1 and Ig-2, each with binding sites for one of the epitopes.

SAQ 22

(a) The antiserum precipitates intact antigen X by cross-linking the molecules as shown in Figure Q7 (the shapes of epitopes 1 and 2 are irrelevant as long as they are different).

(b) Either the peptides do not correspond to epitopes 1 or 2 on the intact antigen, or they do but the antibodies are unable to cross-link adjacent peptides and hence cannot precipitate them from solution.

(c) Excess *loop* peptide inhibits precipitate formation between the antiserum and intact molecules of antigen X, but excess *linear* peptide does not. It follows that the loop peptide must contain an epitope, and that in excess the peptide competes successfully with the intact molecule for binding sites on the antibody. The linear peptide does not compete and therefore does not contain an epitope.

(d) The loop conformation must be essential to the 'fit' between the epitope and the binding sites on the antibody; even though the linear peptide has the *same* amino acid sequence as the loop, the residues do not take up the correct conformation without the stabilising effect of the disulphide bond.

(e) The fact that the loop peptide contains an epitope (as demonstrated by experiment D) but still cannot form a precipitate with the antiserum indicates that it is *monovalent* for the epitope, i.e. it must contain either epitope 1 *or* epitope 2 but not both. (If you are unclear about why the loop must be *monovalent*, look again at Figure Q7; if the loop contained *both* epitopes it would precipitate just as the intact antigen does.) The epitope in the loop occupies the binding sites of the appropriate species of antibody, but no more than two peptides can be linked by the same antibody molecule.

SAQ 23

The amino acids are grouped according to a certain characteristic feature of their side chains: group 1 amino acids have side chains that carry a *charge*; the members of group 2 have large *aromatic* ring structures in their side chains; and group 3 amino acids have side chains that are *neither* charged *nor* aromatic (in fact one has an amide and the other has an hydroxyl group as its side chain). The Table shows that the epitopes in this antigen have a very high proportion of charged or aromatic amino acids in their structure — of 16 residues, only three are neither charged nor aromatic. This suggests that charged and aromatic residues have a particular role in the non-covalent interaction between an epitope and its complementary recognition molecule (antibody or T cell antigen receptor). Charged residues are particularly likely to occur in epitopes because the charge that they carry participates in *ionic bonding* between the epitope and the antigen binding site. Aromatic residues are common because they enter into strong *hydrophobic bonds* with complementary residues, and because the ring structure is a prominent feature in the *shape* of the epitope. All these features contribute to the *specificity* of the interaction between a particular epitope and a particular recognition molecule.

SAQ 24

The answers are given in Table Q5.

TABLE Q5   Blood transfusion combinations

Blood group of donor	Blood group of recipient	Transfusion reaction
A	B	+
B	AB	−
O	A	−
AB	B	+
A	O	+

The reason for transfusion reactions occurring in the combinations indicated in Table Q5 is that the *recipient* in each case has antibodies in their serum that bind to blood group antigens on the *donated* red cells. Transfusion reactions do not occur in the absence of these antibodies, and you can discount the existence of antibodies in the *donor's* serum because they are diluted to such an extent by the recipient's serum.

SAQ 25

You would produce a polyclonal anti-human-IgG antiserum by injecting human IgG into another species, for example a rabbit, and then collecting serum after an immune response has had time to develop. Human IgG heavy chains have certain well defined epitopes that are immunogenic in other species. There are several reasons why a polyclonal antiserum is reasonably easy to produce in this case. First, the antigen (human IgG) is readily available in high concentrations from human peripheral blood; second, responder animals are also readily available; and third, it is relatively simple to adsorb contaminating antibodies from the rabbit antiserum by passing it down an immunoaffinity chromatography column to which human immunoglobulins of all classes *except* IgG have been covalently-linked.

SAQ 26

The answer to this question depends on the fact that the binding interaction between antigen and antibody is a dynamic process (Chapter 6), so the molecules are constantly associating and dissociating. At first, antibodies are in excess of antigen; both remain in solution because the toxin molecules are widely dispersed, all the available epitopes are bound by antibodies, and very few molecules of toxin are cross-linked into immune complexes that are dense enough to precipitate out of solution (as in Figure 7.2a). Then, as antigen concentration rises, more and more molecules of toxin are packed together and more opportunities for cross-linking by antibodies arise; at the equivalence point, the lattices of antigen and antibody become large enough to precipitate out of solution (Figure 7.2b). Finally, as antigen concentration continues to rise still further, the precipitate gradually *dissolves* because too few binding sites on the antibodies are available to cross-link so many molecules of antigen (Figure 7.2c).

SAQ 27

Your graph should look like Figure Q8. There are two conclusions: first that antigen concentration is *proportional* to ring diameter squared; and second that although very dilute concentrations of antigen reach maximum ring diameter after 16 hours, as antigen concentration *increases* so too does the time taken for the antigen to diffuse far enough from the well to reach the equivalence point. This underlines a disadvantage of RID assays for estimating the concentration of antigen samples: they are slow in reaching a stable end-point.

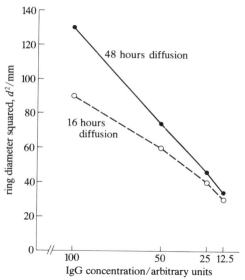

FIGURE Q8 Standard curves of human IgG concentration plotted against ring diameter squared after 16 or 48 hours diffusion in a radial immunodiffusion (RID) assay. (Data from Table Q4 in SAQ 27.)

A d^2 reading of 68 mm converts to an IgG concentration of 46 units on the standard curve plotted from data obtained after 48 hours diffusion. (If you used the curve plotted after only 16 hours diffusion you would obtain an artificially *high* value for IgG concentration.)

SAQ 28

(a) Immunoelectrophoresis takes place under non-denaturing conditions and separates protein antigens on the basis of differences in their net *charge*. Immunoblotting also separates protein antigens by electrophoresis, but in an SDS-containing gel, which denatures the antigens and imparts a strong negative charge to them, so that they separate on the basis of differences in their *mass*.

(b) In immunoelectrophoresis, the separated antigens are identified by allowing specific antibodies to diffuse towards them from a trough cut in the gel. Precipitin lines form at the equivalence points and these may be made more visible by staining. In immunoblotting, the separated antigens are transferred to nitrocellulose paper by applying a second electric current at right angles to the first. Identification involves 'developing' the antigen blots by treating them with radioactively-labelled or enzyme-labelled antibodies or, more often, *un*labelled specific antibodies followed by labelled second antibodies or labelled protein A.

SAQ 29

The plastic container (usually a plate with small wells in it) is first coated with rubella virus antigens and then incubated with the person's serum sample. Unbound antibodies are washed off and then the plate is treated with anti-human-immunoglobulin antibodies (raised in another species) that have been linked to a suitable enzyme. The enzyme-linked antibodies bind to the Fc regions of the anti-rubella antibodies, and when a suitable substrate is added a colour change takes place. The amount of coloured product is proportional to the concentration of anti-rubella antibodies in the person's serum. Figure Q9 shows the various layers of antigen, antibodies, enzyme and substrate that are built up during the assay. (An alternative method of indirect labelling would be to use enzyme-labelled protein A.)

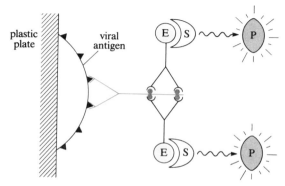

FIGURE Q9 Diagram showing the layers of reagents that interact during an assay for anti-rubella virus antibodies using the ELISA method and indirect labelling. The anti-viral antibodies (red) from the sample of patient's serum bind to solid-phase viral antigen. They are detected by the binding of an enzyme-linked second antibody (E), which acts on a substrate (S) to produce a coloured product (P).

SAQ 30

New-born babies have far fewer mature immunocompetent cells (innate and adaptive) than adults, and their production of antibodies and complement is also much lower. Adult levels are not achieved until at least two years of age. In addition, babies have no memory cells in their circulation because (ideally) they will not have encountered any antigens while in the protection of the uterus. For both these reasons, the immune response of a baby to a new antigen will be relatively slow to develop and may be ineffective. Passively acquired antibodies from colostrum and breast milk are therefore an important source of protection against infection, together with maternal antibodies that crossed the placenta and persist for a few months after birth (see Figure 8.1).

SAQ 31

Thymocytes (immature T cells) migrate through the thymus from cortex to medulla, adhering closely to the long dendritic processes of thymic epithelial cells. These processes are rich in self-MHC molecules. Thymocytes proliferate very rapidly during migration through the cortex, but many die before they reach the medulla. Two models for the self-MHC restriction of the survivor population have been proposed: either thymocytes with TcR chains that bind to self-MHC molecules on the thymic epithelial cells are selected for further maturation, or thymocytes with TcR chains that do *not* bind to self-MHC molecules are selectively destroyed.

SAQ 32

Figure Q4 shows that after challenge with a second immunogenic dose of epitope X (on B1355) the number of plasma cells producing antibodies to epitope X declines with the amount of B512 injected on day one; there is a significant reduction in group B compared with group A (the controls), and an even greater reduction in group C. This indicates that high-zone tolerance to epitope X was induced by the injection of B512. This tolerance is specific for epitope X; all three groups of mice produce similar levels of antibody to epitope Y *even though* it is on the same antigen (B1355) as epitope X in the challenging injection on day 14. Thus, high-zone tolerance induction affects a single clone of B cells—those with receptors for epitope X. (Note that this experiment cannot distinguish between *deletion* of this B cell clone and lack of specific T cell help for it.)

SAQ 33

Inducers of suppression activate suppressor T cells, which in turn inhibit the activity of helper T cells and other types of effector cell (e.g. B cells and macrophages). Inducers of help activate all effector cells *except* suppressor T cells. Contrasuppressors counteract the inhibitory activity of suppressor T cells on helper T cells, i.e. they *reactivate* helper T cells that have been inhibited by suppressor T cells. (A fourth functional subset of helper T cells is involved in delayed hypersensitivity reactions, as you will discover in Chapter 10.)

SAQ 34

The first way is by activating the correct clone of inducers of suppression, which in turn activate the clone of suppressor T cells that have receptors for epitopes on the same antigen as the B cell clone. [There is considerable dispute about the existence of antigen-specific suppressor (and helper) factors in regulatory networks as described here; they may be able to achieve functional specificity by the expression of receptors for lymphokines only on those cells involved in the network (i.e. in contact with antigen).] The second way is through the idiotype network. Even though this network is antigen-independent it is possible to achieve antigen-specific suppression if surface immunoglobulin on cells of the appropriate B cell clone has a *private* idiotope *inside* its antigen binding site. An anti-idiotype clone of suppressor T cells could then act on the B cell clone in an antigen-specific way. The interaction would be between the anti-idiotype and the surface immunoglobulin. Note, that in this case the anti-idiotype may be an 'internal image' of the antigen because it fits into the B cell receptor's binding site for antigen.

SAQ 35

(a)   They would all be T cells of the $H-2^d$ type, some of which would have receptors for antigen Q and would therefore be undergoing clonal expansion and differentiation. The reason they were all T cells is that the initial radiation killed all the animal's immune cells and stem cells, and the mouse was reconstituted with thymus cells that were already committed to differentiate into T cells.

(b)   They would all be B cells of the $H-2^k$ type, because all the T cells had been lysed by treatment with anti-T cell antibodies and complement.

(c)   Yes. Even if it had not been irradiated, the new host would not mount an immune response against the transplanted cells because both sets of MHC molecules are found on the cells of the host (it is a hybrid of $H-2^d$ and $H-2^k$).

(d)   Nothing! Even though the mouse has been reconstituted with T cells and B cells that have previously been exposed to antigen Q, they cannot cooperate with each other to elicit an immune response because they have different $H-2$ haplotypes. The MHC molecules coded for by alleles in the *I region* influence immune responsiveness in part by restricting the cooperation of T and B cells to those that share the same *Ir* genes.

SAQ 36

You may have thought of two problems that must be overcome before an effective vaccine is developed. First, the virus already elicits an antibody response, but this is not protective (presumably because antibody binding to the viral epitope does not interfere with the ability of the virus to bind to CD4 on the target cell); so an effective vaccine must elicit an immune response directed against epitopes that *do* interfere with the replication of the virus, even though these epitopes are not naturally immunogenic in humans. Second, even if an effective vaccine could be developed, the virus is undergoing genetic drift so that the antigens it expresses today may be altered in the future and current vaccines could become useless. The problems facing drug development are, if anything, even more daunting because once a person is infected with HIV, the genetic material of the virus is spliced into the host cell DNA. (This is no different from the mode of replication of any virus and partly explains why we have so few effective treatments for viral infections.)

SAQ 37

The mothers have circulating autoantibodies, in one case to the receptors for thyroid stimulating hormone on thyroid cells, and in the other to acetylcholine receptors on muscle end-plates. The fact that these babies show transient symptoms of their mother's disease should lead you to conclude that the autoantibodies are of the IgG class. They cross the placenta into the foetus and cause symptoms in the days following birth. The baby does not have self-reactive B cells, so the symptoms disappear as the maternal autoantibodies are degraded. (Note that the autoantibodies in thyrotoxicosis are *stimulatory*, whereas those in myasthenia gravis are *destructive*.)

SAQ 38

The antigens of some parasites provoke the synthesis of IgE, and hence may be damaged by type I reactions based on IgE-mediated degranulation of mast cells in the area surrounding the parasite. Multicellular parasites are too large to be engulfed and may persist in the body for long periods in one location, so they may provoke a type II reaction, i.e. antibody-dependent (IgG or IgM) cell-mediated cytotoxicity. In this reaction antibodies form a bridge between the cells of the parasite and innate effector cells (large granular lymphocytes, eosinophils and phagocytes), which externalise their lysosomes on to the parasite's surface. Some parasites have evolved antigen-shedding as a means of escape (Chapter 5); this can lead to type III reactions, in which inflammation is triggered by large amounts of immune complex formed by parasite antigens and the antibodies directed against them. Finally, many parasites are able to survive indefinitely, setting up the chronic cell-mediated reactions seen in type IV granulomas.

OPTIONAL FURTHER READING

Titles in the 'Practical Approach' series published by IRL Press (see below) are particularly recommended to students who use, or intend to use, immunological techniques at work and wish to expand their expertise.

Brown, J. (ed) (1987) *Human Monoclonal Antibodies: a practical approach*, IRL Press.

Catty, D. (ed) (1988) *Antibodies, Volume I: a practical approach*, and (1989) *Antibodies, Volume II: a practical approach*, IRL Press.

Clemens, M. J., Morris, A. G. and Gearing, A. J. H. (eds) (1987) *Lymphokines and Interferons: a practical approach*, IRL Press.

Cohen, I. R. (1988) 'The self, the world and autoimmunity' in *Scientific American*, April 1988, **258**, No. 4, 34–42.

Grange, J. M., Fox, A. and Morgan, N. L. (eds) (1987) *Immunological Techniques in Microbiology*, Society for Applied Bacteriology and Blackwell Scientific Publications.

Klaus, G. G. B. (ed) (1987) *Lymphocytes: a practical approach*, IRL Press.

Male, D., Champion, B. and Cooke, A. (1987) *Advanced Immunology*, Gower Medical Publishing.

Marrack, P. and Kappler, J. (1987) 'The T cell receptor' in *Science*, 20 November 1987, **238**, 1073–9.

Mayer, R. J. and Walker, J. H. (1987) *Immunochemical Methods in Cell and Molecular Biology*, Academic Press.

Playfair, J. H. L. (1987) *Immunology at a Glance* (4th edition), Blackwell Scientific Publications.

Roitt, I. (1988) *Essential Immunology* (6th edition), Blackwell Scientific Publications.

Roitt, I., Brostoff, J. and Male, D. (1985) *Immunology*, Gower Medical Publishing. (Look out for a new edition published by Churchill Livingstone in late 1989 or early 1990.)

Rosen, F., Steiner, L. and Unanue, E. (1988) *Macmillan Dictionary of Immunology*, Macmillan Publishing.

Scientific American (single-topic issue, Oct 1988) 'What science knows about AIDS', **259**, No. 4.

Sikora, K. and Smedley, H. M. (1984) *Monoclonal Antibodies*, Blackwell Scientific Publications.

Williams, A. F. and Barclay, A. N. (1988) 'The immunoglobulin superfamily—domains for cell surface recognition' in *Annual Review of Immunology*, **6**, 381–405.

Williamson, A. R. and Turner, M. W. (1987) *Essential Immunogenetics*, Blackwell Scientific Publications.

Young, D-E. and Cohn, Z. A. (1988) 'How killer cells kill', in *Scientific American*, January 1988, **258**, No. 1, 28–34.

In addition, many articles about the theory and practice of immunology, written in language that should be accessible to you after studying Book 5, can be found in the monthly journal *Immunology Today*, published by Elsevier Science Publishing; the bi-monthly journal *Current Opinion in Immunology*, published by Current Science; and several times a year in the monthly journal *Scientific American*. The simplest way to keep up to date with developments in AIDS research is by consulting the Royal Society of Medicine's bi-monthly newsheet, *The AIDS Letter*, or the weekly journal *New Scientist*, which has a regular section entitled 'AIDS Monitor'.

INDEX

Entries and page numbers in bold type refer to key words.

2,4-dinitrophenol (2,4-DNP), 47
α-foetoprotein, 98
α-helix, 60, 61
acquired immune deficiency syndrome (AIDS), 6, 72, **134**–6, 137
   biology of HIV, 135
   routes of infection, 136
   symptoms, 135
actin-myosin filament, 14
active site, 29
acute inflammatory reaction, **16**, **18**, 19, 28, 29, 50, 52, 140–1
acute phase proteins, 14, **17**, 19
adaptive immunity, 6–9, 12–13, 20–39, 40, 70, 71
   antigen specificity, 20–1, 26
   immunological memory, 8, 9, **22**
   leukocytes, 8, **12**, 20–7, 30–9
   maturation, 111–18
   molecules involved in antigen recognition, 40–67
   primary response, 9, 22–3, 27–8, 50, 59, 82, 124, 153, 154
   regulation, 123–31
   secondary response, 9, 22–3, 27–8, 48, 59, 124, 153
   tolerance, **118**–22
ADCC *see* antibody-dependent cell-mediated cytotoxicity
adrenal axis, **130**, 131
   see also hormones
adrenalin, 141
adrenocorticotropic hormone (ACTH), 130, 131
affinity, 47, 58, 78–81, 90, 94, 113–4
   estimation, 78–81
   of antibodies for antigens, 58, 78–81, 90, 94, 113–14
   labelling, 47
affinity constant (K), **79**
   estimation for antibody–antigen interactions, 79–81, 82
affinity maturation, **58**
agammaglobulinaemia, 148, 154
agglutination
   of soluble antigen, 51, 87, 90, 92
   test for cell-bound antigen, **98**, 99
   see also cross-linking
aggregates (of antigen), 43, 50
   see also cross-linking
AIDS *see* acquired immune deficiency syndrome
allele (of *MHC* genes), 32, 64, 129
allelic exclusion, **53**, 149
allergen, 18, 52, **102**, 121, 132, 140, 141
   airborne, 18, 52, 102, 140
   in food, 18, 52, 140

systemic, 141
allergic inflammatory reaction, 18, 52, 140
allergy, 18, 52, **102**, 121, 134, 141
allogeneic antigens, 85–7, 121
allosteric inhibition, 29
amino acid sequence *see* primary structure
anaemia, 87, 140, 142, 145
ankylosing spondylitis, 139, 140
anthrax, 73
anti-anti-idiotype (antibodies or receptors), 127, **128**
anti-idiotype (antibodies or receptors), 52, 66, **126**, 127, 128, 134, 158
anti-immunoglobulin antibodies, 100, 102, 156
antibiotic, 142
antibody, 8, **25**
   action of secreted antibodies, 28–9
   in ADCC, **16**, 19, 28, 29, 141, 142
   affinity for antigen, 58, 78–81, 90, 94, 113–14
   affinity maturation, **58**
   agglutination of antigen, 51, 87, 90, 92
   aggregation of antigen, 43, 50
   antigen binding site, **20**, 25, 42–3
   antigen recognition, 48
   antigen specificity, 20–1, 26, 52–3, 90, 92, 94
   anti-anti-idiotype, 127, **128**
   anti-idiotype, 52, 66, **126**, 127, 128, 134, 158
   anti-immunoglobulin (second antibodies), 100, 102, 156
   anti-Rhesus, 87
   applications in laboratory assays, 89, 90, 92, 94–107
   as an opsonin, 14, 28, 29, 49, 154
   autoantibodies, 89, 106, **121**, 142, 145, 158, Plates 8.1, 10.1 and 10.2
   classes, 44, **48**–52
      (*see also* IgA, IgD, IgE, IgG *and* IgM)
   class switching, 58, **59**, 82, 113, 124, 154
   complement activation, 28, 29, 49
   concentration effects on immune response, 124
   constant domain, **44**, 48, 49, 50, 51
   constant region, **43**–4, 48, 54
   cross-linking of antigens, 43, 50, 51, 76, 79, 81, 90, 92, 95
   cross-reacting, 82, 83, 84, 108
   diagnostic uses, 97, 98, 102, 106, 107, 108, 109
   estimation of *K* (affinity constant), 79–81
   Fab region, 25, **26**, **41**–2, 81, 149
   Fc region, 25, **26**, **41**–2, 99, 108, 149
   flexibility, 43, 51

genes *see* immunoglobulin genes
heavy chain, **41**, 42, 43, 44, 46, 47, 48, 53, 55, 56–7, 112, 113
hinge region, **42**
history of research, 40–1
hypervariable loops, **44**, 45, 46, 47, 108
   in **immune complexes**, **79**, 91, 95, 96, 100, 140, 142, 146, 157
J-chain, **50**, 51
kappa:lambda ratio, 54
kappa light chain and genes, **53**–4, 55, 56
lag phase, 27, 28
lambda light chain, **53**–4
levels in foetus and new-born, 111, 112
light chain, **41**, 42, 43, 44, 45, 46, 47
monoclonal (Mabs), 40, **92**–4, 106, 108, 109, 110, 134, 137
   in **polyclonal antiserum**, 81, 90, **91**–2, 94, 98, 151
   polymerisation, 48, 49, 50, 51
   precipitation of soluble antigen, 90, 92, 95, 150, 156
   primary response, **9**, 27–8, 50, 59, 82, 124
   purification by **immunoaffinity chromatography**, **91**, 156
   relative molecular mass (M_r), 49
   repertoire, 52
   secondary response, **9**, 22–3, 27–8, 48, 59, 124
   secretion, 25, 50
   secretory piece, **50**
   serum concentration and half-life, 49
   somatic mutation, **58**
   somatic recombination, **55**–9, 112, 149
   species, 81
   structural domains, 43, 49
   structure (primary and higher-order), 25–6, **41**–8
   subclasses, 48
   supergene family, 67, **68**
   surface immunoglobulin (sIg), **25**–6, 31, 50, 58, 76, 106, 112–3
   therapeutic uses *in vivo*, 108, 109, 110
   in transfusion reactions to ABO antigens, 86–7, 150–1, 156
   valency, 48, 49, 50, 51, 90, 113–4, 149, 155
   variable recombination, **57**–8
   variable domain, **44**, 45
   variable region, **43**–4, 45, 46, 47, 49, 50, 51, 54
   VDJ cluster or combination, 55, 56, 57, 58
antibody-dependent cell-mediated cytotoxicity (ADCC), **16**, 19, 28, 29, 141, 142
antibody-dependent cytotoxic hypersensitivity (type II), **141**–2

Goodpasture's syndrome, 139, 142,
 Plate 10.1
 haemolytic anaemia, 142
 myasthenia gravis, 139, 142
antibody–hapten complex, 79
antibody-independent cytotoxicity, 15
antigen, 8, 20
 2,4-dinitrophenol (2,4-DNP), 47
 α-foetoprotein, 98
 aggregates, agglutinates or lattices, 28,
  29, 43, 50, 51, 87, 95
 affinity for antibody, 58, 78–81 90, 94,
  113–14
 allogeneic, **85**–7, 121
 antigenic cells or molecules, **46**–7
 antigenic drift, **74**, 158
 antigenic shift, **74**
 blood group (ABO), **86**–7
 carcinoembryonic, 67, 68, 137
 charged residues, 78, 156
 concentration effects on immune
  response, 123
 conformation, 84, 85
 cross-linking by antibodies, 43, 50, 51,
  76, 79, 81, 82, 90, 92, 95
 cross-reacting, **82**, **83**, 84
 denatured, 84
 detection or quantification in
  laboratory assays, 95–107
 differentiation, **88**
 disguise by parasites, 75
 embryonic, **88**
 epitope, **8**, 10, 20, 21, 76–7, 84, 85
 estimation of K (affinity constant),
  79–81
 flexibility of bond angles, 79
 'foreignness', 78, 88
 glycolipid, 8, 76
 glycoprotein, 8, 76
 haemagglutinin, 84, 85
 hapten, **46**–7, 76, 79, 80, 81, 83, 89
 hapten–carrier conjugate or complex,
  47, 76, 89
 hydrophobic residues, 78, 156
 idiotope, 52, 66, 117, **126**, 127, 128, 134
 in **immune complexes**, **79**, 91, 95, 96,
  100, 140, 142, 146, 157
 immunogenic cells or molecules, **46**–7,
  52, 76, 85, 138
 leukocyte, 106
 lipid, 76
 monovalent, 79
 multivalent, 76, 81, 82, 90, 92, 95
 native (intact), 26, 84
 nickel, 76, 143, 144
 oligosaccharide, 76
 oncofoetal, **137**
 penicillin, 76, 85
 polymers, 26, 27, 76, 155
 polypeptide, 8, 84
 polysaccharide, 17, 27, 76, 151
 processing, **33**, 47, 84, 85
 protein, 76–9
 purification by **immunoaffinity**

chromatography, **91**, 94–5
 range of, 10
 Rhesus, 86, **87**
 self-epitope, **118**, 119, 128, 139, 142, 145
 size, 45–6, 76
 sperm whale myoglobin, 77
 structure, 76–7
 T cell-dependent, **26**, 27, 153
 T cell-independent, **26**, 27, 75, 76, 153
 tissue-specific, 87–**88**
 transplantation, 60, 86, 109
 tumour-specific, 108, 109, 137
 in vaccines, 9, 135–6
 valency, 76, 79, 81, 82, 90, 92, 95
 xenogeneic, 85, 87–8
antigen binding site, **20**, 25, 42–3, 60–1,
  62, 65, 66, 67
 on antibody molecules, 20, 25, 42
 on MHC molecules, 60–1, 62
 on TcR chains, 65, 66, 67
antigen-driven maturation, **112**
 of B cells, 113, 114
 of T cells, 34
antigen-independent maturation, 112
 of B cells, 112, 113
 of T cells, 114–8
antigen presenting cell (APC), 32, **33**, 37,
  70, 67, 85, 120, 125, 126
 B cell, 33
 dendritic cell, **33**, 37, 70
 macrophage, 33, 37, 70
 role in regulating immune response,
  125–6
 role in self-tolerance, 120
 traffic through lymphoid system, 37
antigen processing, **33**, 47, 84, 85
antigen receptor, **20**–1
 diversity of, 21
 on B cells, **25**–6, 31, 50 106, 112–3
 on **T cells**, **31**, 41, 65–6, 106
antigen specificity, **20**–1
 of antibodies, 26, 52–3
 of monoclonal antibodies, 92, 94
 of polyclonal antisera, 90
 of T cells, 65
antigenic cells or molecules, **46**–7
 see also **immunogenic**
antigenic drift, **74**, 158
antigenic shift, **74**
antiserum, **81**
 polyclonal, 90, 91–2, 94, 98
antisome, 7, 8
arthritic disease, 139–40, 146, 147
 ankylosing spondylitis, 139, 140
 association with *HLA* alleles, 139, 140
 post-infection arthritis, 139
 Reiter's disease, 139
 rheumatoid arthritis, 139, 146, 147
artificial **tolerance** induction, 120–1, 151
 high-zone, **121**, 134, 157
 low-zone, **121**
Ascaris lumbricoides, 75
assembled epitope, 76, 77
associative recognition, **66**, 84–5, 129

autoantibody, 89, 106, **121**, 142, 145, 158,
  Plates 8.1, 10.1 and 10.2
autocrine stimulation of helper T cells,
  124
autoimmune disease, 88, 89, 106, 118, **121**,
  122, 129, 130, 132, 134, 142, **145**, 146
 Addison's disease, 139
 association with *HLA* alleles, 139
 chronic active hepatitis, 139
 dermatitis herpetiformis, 139
 Goodpasture's syndrome, 139, 142,
  Plate 10.1
 haemolytic anaemia, 142
 Hashimoto's thyroiditis, 139, 146
 insulin-dependent diabetes, 139
 male infertility, 145
 multiple sclerosis, 139
 myasthenia gravis, 139, 142, 152, 158
 non-organ specific (generalised), 146
 organ-specific, 139, 145, 146
 pernicious anaemia, 145
 premature menopause, 145
 rheumatoid arthritis, 139, 146, 147
 Sjögren's syndrome, 139
 systemic lupus erythematosus, 139, 146,
  Plate 10.2
 thyrotoxicosis, 139, 146, 152, 158
avidity, 81, **82**, 90, 94

B cell, **8**, **22**–4, **25**–7
 activation, 26–7, 35
 antigen recognition, 25–6
 as an antigen-presenting cell, 33
 Bursa of Fabricius, 23–4
 congenital immune deficiency, 133
 development, 13, 23–4, 111–4
 epitopes, 76, 77, **84**–5
 immature, 112, 118
 in lymphoid organs, 37, 39
 mature, 22–3, 111, 112, 113
 memory, 24, 28, 111, 113
 naive, **22**–3, 111, 112, 113
 plasma cell, **25**, 39, 52, 92, 108, 113, 154
 plasmacytoma, 92
 polyclonal activation, 27, 75, 135
 pre-B, 112, 114
 self-reactive, 118, 119, 120, 121, 122,
  145, 158
 surface immunoglobulin, **25**–6, 31, 50,
  58, 76, 106, 112–3
 traffic through lymphoid and vascular
  system, 36–9, 154
B cell plaque-forming assay, **107**, 108
B lymphocyte, **8**, **22**
 see also B cell
β-pleated sheet, 44, 60–1
$β_2$-microglobulin, **60**, 62, 155
bacteria, 5
 escape strategies, 11, 73–4
 immune response to, 9, 14, 17, 18, 19,
  27, 28, 29, 71, 133, 153
 sugars in cell walls, 14, 17, 78, 86, 153
basement membrane, 14, 19

basophil, 13, **16**, 19, 49, 51
binding site *see* antigen binding site
bioassays, 108
Bjorkman, P., 41
blood group antigens (ABO), **86**-7
    blood typing, 86
blotting methods *see* immunoblotting
bond angle (flexibility of), 79
bone marrow, 12, 24, 36-7, 39, 109, 116, 133
    grafting, 133
bovine serum albumin (BSA), 47
breakdown of self-tolerance, 121-2
bronchospasm/dilation, 141
Brucella abortus, 111
brucellosis, 72, 111
bubonic plague, 72
Burkitt's lymphoma, 27
Bursa of Fabricius, 23-4
bystander damage, 34, 108

C- and N-termini (of polypeptides), 42, 45
c-myc, 138
C3a, C3b, and C5a *see* complement
cancers, 88, 106, 108
    Burkitt's lymphoma, 27
    diagnosis, 108, 109
    immune surveillance theories, 136-8
    Kaposi sarcoma, 135, 137
    leukaemias, 106, 109, 137, 138
    lymphomas, 27, 106, 138
    malignant transformation, 137-8
    myelomas, 92, 138
    plasmacytoma, 92
    solid-tissue, 137
    therapy, 108, 133, 134, 136-8
carbohydrate residues
    in antibody heavy chains, 48
    in bacterial cell walls, 14, 17, 78, 86
    in epitopes, 45
carcinoembryonic antigen (CEA), 67, 68, 137
carrier molecule, 46, 47
cascade reaction *see* complement
CD molecule (cluster of differentiation), 30, 31
    CD2, 31, 67, 68, 107, 114
    CD3 complex, 31, 65, **66**, 67, 68, 117, 155
    CD4, 31, 64, 67, 68, 106, 107, 114, 117, 135, 148, 153, 158
    CD8, 31, 66, 67, 68, 106, 107, 114, 117
    CD11, 31
cDNA, 66
cell-mediated immunity, **24**, 111
cell-mediated hypersensitivity *see* delayed hypersensitivity
Chagas disease, 74
chemotactic factor, **18**, 19, 34, 35, 70, 148, 153
    C5a, 18, 19
    secreted by macrophages, 19, 70

secreted by mast cells, 18, 19
secreted by helper T cells, 34, 35
chickenpox (rubella), 148, 153, 157
chromatography, 91
    see also immunoaffinity chromatography
cilia, 11, 12
circadian rhythms in immune responsiveness, 131
class I MHC molecules, **32**, 33, **60**, 61, 63, 66-7, 86, 117, 129, 148, 155
    genes, 63, 129
    expression, 32
    interaction with CD8, 66-7
    role in self-MHC restriction, 117
    structure, 60-1
class II MHC molecules, **32**, 33, **61-2**, 63, 67, 70, 117, 129, 139, 149
    genes, 63, 129, 139
    expression, 32, 70
    interaction, with CD4, 67
    role in self-MHC restriction, 117
    structure, 61-2
class switching *see* immunoglobulin class switching
clonal abortion model of self-tolerance, 118, **119**, 120
clonal expansion, **22**, 23, 28, 113, 114
clonal selection, **21**, 23
clone *see* lymphocyte clone
cloning of cells and genes, 40, 92
clotting factors, 18
co-evolution, 72
coagulase, 73
collaboration between innate and adaptive immunity, 7, 16, 17, 28, 29, 33, 34, 35, 39, 70, 71
colostrum, 50, 112, 151, 157
common cold virus, 150, 155
competitive inhibition assays, 101, 102, 103
complement, **17**-8, 19, 28, 29, 63, 64, 71, 108, 129
    activation by bound antibody, 28, 29, 49, 71
    cascade reaction, 17, 28, 29, 41, 49, 50, 70, 71, 74, 140, 149, 153, 154
    components
        C3a, 18, 19, 73
        C3b, 18, 19, 111, 133, 153, 154
        C5a, 18, 19, 73, 153, 154
    genes, 63, 64
    genetic abnormality, 129
    membrane attack complex, **18**, 19, 28, 29, 154
    opsonisation, **14**, 18, 19, 28, 29, 50, 111, 153
    use in assays, 108, 148, 149
computer modelling, 48
conformation of antibodies and antigens, 84, 85
conformational change, 29, 78
congenic strain, **64**, 115, 149, 155
congenital immune deficiency, **133**

constant
    domain, **44**, 48, 49, 50, 51, 65, 68
    region, **43**-4, 48, 54
    region genes (*C*), 54, 55, 56, 57, 58, 59
contact hypersensitivity, 143, 144
contrasuppressor cell, **125**, 151, 158
cornea, 72
Corynebacterium diphtheriae, 29
cowpox, 83, 153
cross-linking
    of B cell antigen-receptors, 26, 27, 76, 128
    of cell-bound antigen, 98, 99
    of soluble antigen, 43, 50, 51, 76, 79, 81, 82, 90, 92, 95
cross-reaction, 44, 82, **83**, 84, 108, 121
    in breakdown of self-tolerance, 121
    of antibodies, 82, 83, 84, 108
    of antigens, 44, 82, 83, 84
cyclic AMP, 66
    see also signal transduction
cyclosporin A, 121, 134
cytokine, **33**, 34
    interleukin-1 (Il-1), **34**, 35, 70
cytotoxic white cells, 7, **8**, **15**, 19
    eosinophil, 12, 13, 14, **15**, 71
    K cell, **16**, 28
    NK cell, **15**, 16, 17, 19, 35, 71, 130, 136, 148, 153, 155
    T cell, 30, 60, 66, 67, 71, 114, 125, 129, 135, 136, 148, 149, 154, 155
cytotoxicity, 8, 13, 15-6, 17, 18, 19
    antibody-dependent cell-mediated, **16**, 19, 28, 29, 141, 142
    membrane attack complex, **18**, 19, 28, 29, 154
    osmotic pressure effects, 16
    perforin, **15**
cytotoxic drug, 108

D-galactose, 86
D-region see HLA complex
Davis, M., 41
degranulation *see* mast cell
delayed hypersensitivity (type IV), 142-3, 144, 145
    contact, 143, 144
    granulomatous, 143, 145
    tuberculin, 143
delayed hypersensitivity T cell, 30, **142**, 143
denatured
    antibody, 91
    antigen, 47, 84
dendritic cell, **33**, 37, 70
    see also antigen presenting cell
development of immune competence, 111, 112
Di George syndrome, 150, 155
diagnostic uses of antibodies, 97, 98, 102, 106, 107, 108, 109
differentiation antigen, **88**
diffuse lymphoid tissue, 36

dimer (of IgA), **50**, 73, 113, Plate 4.1
diphtheria, 29, 142, 151
direct and indirect labelling methods *see* immunolabelling
disulphide bonding, 44, 45, 48
diurnal rhythms in immune responsiveness, 131
DNA hybridisation, 66
DNA splicing *see* somatic recombination
Doherty, P., 116, 148–9
domain *see* structural domain
downstream and upstream sequences in DNA, 56, 57, 58
dual recognition model of MHC-restriction, 66
dynamic balance between host and pathogen, 72

Edelman, G., 41
effector cells in adaptive immunity, 22, 23, 125
see also B cell and T cell
electroblotting, 104
electron-dense structure, 12
see also granule
electrophoresis, 97, 98, 104
see also immunoelectrophoresis
embryonic antigen, **88**
endemic diseases, 72
endocrine influence on immune responsiveness, 130–1
endorphins, 131
enzyme-labelling methods, 100, 102–4, 105, 106
   enzyme-linked immunosorbent assay (ELISA), **103**, 104, 151, 157
   immunoblotting, **105**
   immunohistochemistry, **106**, Plates 8.1, 10.1 and 10.2
enzyme–substrate interactions, 80, 81
enzymes
   alkaline phosphatase, 102
   anti-HIV, 136
   coagulase, 73
   horse-radish peroxidase, 102, Plate 8.1
   hyaluronidase, 73
   lysozyme, 11, 12, **17**, 19, 71, 73, 150, 153
   papain, 149
   protease, 73
eosinophil, 12, 13, 14, **15**, 71
epidemic, 71
epidermal growth factor, 129
epitope, **8**, 10, 20, 21, 45, 76–9, 84, 85
   assembled, 76, 77
   B cell, 76, 77, **84–5**
   conformation, 84, 85
   diversity, 10, 45
   flexibility of bond angles, 79
   'foreignness', 78
   internal, 76, 77, 84, 85
   linear, 76, 77, 84, 85
   residues, 45, 78, 150

size, 45, 76
structure, 76–9
surface, 76, 77
T cell, 76, 77, **84–5**
valency, 76
Epstein-Barr (EB) virus, 27, 31
equilibrium dialysis, **79**, 80
equivalence point, **95**, 96, 97
   see also precipitin reaction
escape strategies, **72–5**
   bacterial, 11, 73–4
   parasite, 74–5
   viral, 74, 135–6
exon, 55, 68
extracellular chemical defences in innate immunity, 17

Fab region, 25, **26**, **41–2**, 81, 149
Factor VIII, 136
Farmer's lung disease, 142
Fc receptor, 41, 67, 68
   on B or T cells, 31, 124
   on cytotoxic cells, 28, 29, 49
   on mast cells, 49, 71, 140
   on phagocytes, 28, 29, 49, 154
Fc region, 25, **26**, **41–2**, 99, 108, 149
Ficoll density-gradient, 107
filariasis, 145
flexibility
   of antibody molecule, 43, 51
   of bond angles in antigens, 79
fluorescent labelling methods, 90, 106, 107
   flow cytofluorography, **106**, 107
   fluorescence-activated cell sorter (FACS), **107**
   immunofluorescence, **106–7**
   in immunohistochemistry, **106**, Plates 8.1, 10.1 and 10.2
foetal immunity, 111, 112
follicle stimulating hormone (FSH), 145
'foreignness' of an antigen or epitope, 78, 88
functional deletion model of self-tolerance, 118, **119**, 120
fungi, 5, 71, 135

gels in antigen/antibody assays, 95, 96, 97, 98
gene
   pool, 72
   segment, 54
   sequencing, 40
   splicing, 55
generation of diversity
   in antibodies, 53–8
   in MHC molecules, 64
   in TcR chains, 66
genetic engineering, 40, 55, 108
genome, 52, 55, 58, 74, 108, 135
germ-line
   gene, **53**, 54, 55, 66, 111, 149

cell, 53, 54, 55, 66, 149
giant or epithelioid cell, 143
glucocorticoids, 130, 131
glycolipid antigen, 8, 76
glycoprotein antigen, 8, 76
gonorrhoea, 73
Goodpasture's syndrome, 139, 142, Plate 10.1
graft rejection, 7, **8**, 9, 10, 60, 61, 64, 72, 86
graft versus host disease, 109, **110**
Gram-negative bacteria, 74
Gram-positive bacteria, 155
granule, 13, 16
granulocytes, **12**, 13
granuloma, 143, 145
granulomatous hypersensitivity, 143

H-2 complex, **63**, 64, 115, 129
   H-2D region, 115, 116, 152, 158
   H-2K region, 115, 116, 152, 158
   I-region, 63, 64, 129, 158
H-substance, 86
haemagglutination, 99
haemagglutinin, 84, 85
haemoglobin, 87
haemolytic anaemia (autoimmune), 142
haemolytic disease of the new-born, 87
haemophilia, 136
Haemophilus influenzae, 73
half-life of antibodies, 49, 87
haplotype, 115
hapten, **46**–7, 76, 79, 80, 81, 83, 89
   2,4-dinitrophenol, 47
hapten–carrier conjugate or complex, 47, 76, 89, 149, 154
Hashimoto's thyroiditis, 139, 146
heavy chain, **41–8**, 53, 55–7, 112, 113
   genes (*V, D, J, C*), 53, 54, 55, 57, 58, 59
   structure, 41–8, 53, 55–7, 112, 113
helper factor *see* lymphokines
helper T cell, **30**–1, 33–5, 62, 66–7, 107, 114, 124–8, 130–1, 135, 142–3, 151, 158
   class II MHC-restriction, 62, 66, 67, 114, 149
   contrasuppressor cell, **125**, 151, 158
   delayed hypersensitivity cell, **30**, 142, 143
   helper : suppressor ratio, 107, 135
   inducer of help, **125**, 151, 158
   inducer of suppression, **125**, 151, 158
   interleukin-2 receptor density, 124–5
   lymphokine secretion, **34–5**, 123, 125, 128, 130, 131, 143, 154
   role in idiotype networks, 127, **128**
   role in regulating immune response, 30–1, 33–5, 107, 125–6, 135
   susceptibility to HIV infection, 135
hen egg-white lysozyme, 150
high endothelial venule, 37, 38, Plate 3.2
high-zone tolerance, **121**, 134, 157
higher-order structure
   of antibodies, 25–6, 41–8

higher-order structure—*cont.*
  of antigens, 76–7
  of immunoglobulin superfamily, 67–8
  of MHC molecules, 60–2
  of T cell antigen receptor, 65–6
hinge region of antibody molecule, **42**
histamine, 16
HIV *see* human immunodeficiency virus
HLA complex, **63**, 64, 129, 138, 139, 140,
  145
  D-region, 63, 64, 129, 139, 140
  HLA-associated diseases, 138, 139, 140
  major gene loci (*A, B, C, DP, DQ, DR*),
    63, 64
hormones
  adrenal axis, **130**, 131
  adrenocorticotropic hormone (ACTH),
    130, 131
  cytokines, 33
  follicle stimulating hormone (FSH),
    145
  glucocorticoids, 130, 131
  growth hormone, 130
  hypothalamic releasing factors, 130,
    131
  insulin, 129, 130
  lymphokines, 34–5
  oxytocin, 130
  sex hormones, 130
  thymic hormones, 117
  thyroid hormones, 130, 146
  thyroid stimulating hormone (TSH),
    146, 158
host, **5**, 72, 109, 110
  see also graft versus host disease
human immunodeficiency virus (HIV), 6,
  29, 74, 107, **134**, 135, 136, 148, 152, 158
  biology, 134–5
  routes of infection, 136
human serum albumin (HSA), 99
humoral immunity, **24**, 111
hyaluronidase, 73
hybrid strain, 115
hybridoma, **92**, 93
hydrogen bonding, 78
hydrophilic sections of polypeptide, 60,
  61
hydrophobic
  forces or interactions, 60, 78, 156
  groups or residues, 45, 78, 156
  sections of polypeptide, 25, 42, 60
hypersensitivity reactions, 52, **140**–5, 152,
  158
  type I, 140–1
  type II, 141–2, Plate 10.1
  type III, 143, 146, Plate 10.2
  type IV, 142–3, 144, 145
hypervariable loops, **44**, 45, 46, 47, 108
hypothalamic releasing factors, 130
hypothalamus, 34, 130, 131

I-region see H-2 complex
iatrogenic disorders, 132

identical twins, 32, 64
idiopathic disorders, 132
idiotope, **52**, 66, 117, **126**, 127, 128, 134
  private, **126**, 127, 134, 158
idiotype, 52, 66, **126**, 127
  anti-idiotype, 52, 66, **126**, 127, 128, 134,
    158
  anti-anti-idiotype, 127, **128**
idiotype network regulation, 126–**128**, 158
Il-2 and Il-2 receptor *see* interleukin-2
immature B cell, 112, 118
immediate hypersensitivity (type I), **140**–1
  allergy, 18, 52, **102**, 121, 134, 141
immune, **9**, 153
immune cell circuits
  helper : suppressor regulation, 30–1,
    33–5, 107, 125–6, 135
  idiotype network regulation, 126–8,
    158
immune competence, **111**, 112, 145
immune complex, **79**, 91, 95, 96, 100, 140,
  142, 146, 156, 157, Plate 10.2
immune complex-mediated
  hypersensitivity (type III), 142, 146, 152,
    158, Plate 10.2
  Farmer's lung disease, 142
  pigeon fancier's disease, 142
  serum sickness, 142
  systemic lupus erythematosus, 146,
    Plate 10.2
immune deficiency, **132**–6
  congenital, 133, 148, 154, 150, 155
  induced, 133–6
immune hyperactivity, **132**, **138**–46
  autoimmune, 145–6
  congenital, 138–40
  hypersensitivity, 140–5
immune response
  potential of, 10
  to bacteria, 9, 14, 17, 18, 19, 27, 28, 29,
    71, 133, 153
  to fungi, 71
  to parasites, 9, 15, 17–8, 28, 30, 52, 71,
    152, 153, 158, Plate 5.1
  to viruses, 9, 15, 16, 17, 29, 30, 71, 133,
    135–6, 153
immune responsiveness, **111**–2, 123–7, 128,
  129, 130, 131, 132, 139
  circadian and diurnal rhythms, 131
  effect of age, 111–2
  individual variation, 78, 128–9
  Ir genes, **129**, 158
  regulation by antibody and antigen
    concentration, 123–4
  regulation by receptor density, 124–5,
    129
  regulation by idiotype networks, 126–7,
    158
  regulation by immune-cell circuits,
    30–1, 33–5, 107, 125–6, 135
  regulation by neuroendocrine
    mechanisms, 130–1
immune systems
  invertebrate, 6–7

vertebrate, 6–7
immune surveillance theories of cancer,
  136–8
immunoaffinity chromatography, **91**, 94–5,
  156
  of polyclonal antisera, 91, 156
  of antigen mixtures, 94–5
immunoblotting (Western blotting), **104**,
  105, 151, 157
immunodiffusion methods, **96**–7, 98
  Ouchterlony diffusion test, 96
  radial immunodiffusion assay (RID),
    96–7, 151, 156–7
immunoelectrophoresis, **97**–8, 104, 151,
  157
  in **immunoblotting**, **104**–5, 151, 157
  rocket immunoelectrophesis, **98**
immunofluorescence methods, 90, **106**–7
  flow cytofluorography, **106**–7
  fluorescence activated cell sorter, **107**
  in **immunohistochemistry**, **106**, Plates
    8.1, 10.1 and 10.2
immunogenic cells or molecules, **46**–7, 52,
  76, 85, 138
immunoglobulin classes, **44**, 48–52
  class switching, 58, **59**, 82, 113, 124, 154
  IgA, 48, 49, **50**, 59, 71, 73, 111, 112,
    149, 155, Plate 4.1
  IgD, 48, 49, **51**, 58, 154
  IgE, 16, 28, 49, **51**–2, 59, 71, 75, 102,
    140, 141, 158
  IgG, 42, **48**, 49, 59, 71, 82, 87, 90, 97,
    100, 111, 112, 124, 141, 142, 149, 154,
    155, 158
  IgM, 48, 49, **50**, 58–9, 68, 71, 82, 86, 87,
    90, 111, 112, 124, 141, 142, 154, 155,
    Plate 4.2
  subclasses, 48
  surface (sIg), **25**, 31, 50, 106, 112–3
immunoglobulin genes (*V, D, J* and *C*), **52**,
  53, 54, **54**–9, 111, 138
  somatic mutation, **58**
  somatic recombination, **55**–9, 149
  variable recombination, **57**–8
immunoglobulin supergene family, **67**, **68**,
  137
immunohistochemistry, **106**
immunolabelling methods, 99, **100**
  direct labelling, 100
  indirect labelling or sandwich methods,
    100
  with enzymes, 102–4, 105, 106,
    Plates 8.1, 10.1 and 10.2
  with fluorescent compounds, 90, 106,
    107, Plates 8.1, 10.1 and 10.2
  with protein A, 100, 102, 106
  with radioactive compounds, 90, 100,
    102, 108
immunological memory, **8**, 9, **22**
  see also memory cells
immunological tolerance, **118**–22
  artificial induction, 120–1, 134, 151
  critical period, 118
  high-zone, **121**, 134, 157

low-zone, 121
self-tolerance, 9, 51, 86, **118**–20, 121–2, 128
immunopathology, 132–47
  immune deficiency disorders, 132–37
  immune hyperactivity disorders, 138–47
immunosuppression, **133**–6
  antigen-specific, 126, 134, 151
  congenital, 133
  by drugs, 121, 130, 134
  by HIV infection, 135–6
  by ionising radiation, 133
  by neuroendocrine mechanisms, 130–1
  by parasites, 74, 134
  by **suppressor T cells**, 30, 34, 35, 75, 118, 119, 120, 122, 125, 126, 128, 135
  in self-tolerance, 121
immunosuppressive drugs, 121, 130, 134
  cyclosporin A, 121, 134
immunotherapy for cancers, 108, **137**
inducer of help, **125**, 151, 158
  see also helper T cells
inducer of suppression, **125**, 151, 158
  see also helper T cells
infectious diseases caused by microbes, 5
  anthrax, 73
  bubonic plague, 72
  brucellosis, 72, 111
  chickenpox, 148, 153
  common cold, 150, 155
  cowpox, 83
  diphtheria, 29, 142, 151
  gonorrhoea, 73
  influenza, 74, 84, 85, 150
  Legionnaire's disease, 74
  leprosy, 74
  measles, 72, 148, 153
  pneumonia, 27, 111, 135
  rabies, 72
  rickettsia fevers, 74
  sleeping sickness, 74
  smallpox, 83
  tuberculosis, 74
  yellow fever, 72
inflammation, 8
  acute, **16**, **18**, 19, 28, 29, 50, 52, 140–1
  allergic, 18, 52, 140
  chronic, 143
influenza, 74, 84, 85, 150
innate immunity, 6–8, 13–9, 70, 71, 153
insulin, 129, 130
interferons, **17**, 19, 34, 35, 70, 148, 153, 155
interleukins, 34, 35, 70, 108, 124–5
  interleukin-1 (Il-1), **34**, 35, 70, 130, 131
  interleukin-2 (Il-2), 35, 124–5, 129
  interleukin-2 receptor density, 124–5
  Il-3, Il-4, Il-5 and Il-6, 35
internal epitope, 76, 77, 84, 85
internal image of the antigen, **126**, 127, 158
intrinsic factor, 145
intron, 55

invertebrate immune systems, 6–7
ionic bonding, 78, 156
ionising radiation, 133
Ir genes, **129**, 158
isotope see radioactive labelling methods

J-chain, **50**, 51
Jenner, E., 83
Jerne, N., 128

K see affinity constant
K cell, **16**, 28
Kabat, E., 44
Kaposi sarcoma, 135, 137
kappa : lambda ratio, 54
kappa (κ) **light chain** and genes, **53**–4, 55, 56, 149
kidney glomerulus, 142, Plates 10.1 and 10.2
K_m, 80
Köhler, G., 92, 94, 128

lag phase (in antibody response), 27, 28
lambda (λ) **light chain** and genes, **53**–4, 55, 56, 149
large granular lymphocyte, 13, 15, 16
  see also K cell and NK cell
lattice, 28, 29, 95
  see also agglutination, aggregates, immune complex
Legionella pneumophilia, 74
Legionnaire's disease, 74
Leishmania species, 74, 143
lentivirus, 135
leprosy, 74
leukaemias, 106, 109, 137, 138
leukocyte, 8, **12**, 14, 20–7, 30–9, 111
  antigens, 106
  basophil, 13, **16**, 19, 49, 51
  eosinophil, 12, 13, 14, **15**, 71
  granulocyte, **12**, 13
  K cell, 16, 28
  large granular lymphocytes, 13, 15, 16
  lymphoid cell, **12**, 114
  macrophage, 13, **14**, 17, 18, 19, 33, 34, 35, 37, 49, 70, 74, 120, 125, 126, Plates 2.1 and 2.2
  mast cell, 13, **16**, 18, 19, 28, 29, 49, 52, 70, 71, 75, 102, 140, 141, Plate 2.3
  monocyte, **13**
  neutrophil, 12, 13, **14**, 49, 71, 125, Plates 2.1 and 5.1
  NK cell, **15**, 16, 17, 19, 35, 71, 130, 136, 148, 153, 155
  small lymphocyte, 12, **20**, 22, Plates 3.1 and 3.2 (see also B cell and T cell)
ligand, 8, 20, 30
light chain, **41**–7, 53–6
  structure, 41, 42, 43, 44, 45, 46, 47
  genes (*V, J, C*), 53, 54, 55, 56
linear epitope, 76, 77, 84, 85

lipid antigens, 76
low-zone tolerance, **121**
lymphatic circulation, 36–9, 71
lymphoid system, 12, 36–38
  bone marrow, 12, 24, 36, 37, 39, 109, 116
  diffuse lymphoid tissue, 36
  distribution of B and T cells, 37, 39
  lymph, 36
  lymph nodes, 12, 36, 37, 38
  lymphatic capillaries, 12, 36, 37, 38
  lymphatic vessels (afferent and efferent), 36, 37, 38
  peripheral (or secondary) **lymphoid system**, **36**, 37
  primary lymphoid organs, **36**, 37
  spleen, 12, 36, 37, 38
  thymus, 24, 30, 36, 37, 137, 150, 155
  tonsils, 12, 36, 37
  traffic of B and T cells, 37–9
lymphocyte clone, **21**, 22
lymphoid cell, **12**, 114
lymphokines, **34**–5, 123, 125, 128, 130, 131, 143, 154
  antigen-specific helper factors, 35, 125–6
  antigen-specific suppressor factors, 34–5, 125–6, 151
  B cell growth factors (Il-4, Il-5, Il-6), 35
  chemotactic factor, 35
  colony stimulating factor (Il-3), 35
  interferon, **17**, 19, 34, 35, 70, 148, 153, 155
  interleukin-2 (Il-2), 35, 124–5
  lymphotoxin, 35
  macrophage activation factor (MAF), 35
  migration inhibition factor (MIF), 35
lymphomas, 106, 138
lysosome, 14, 28, 74, 141
lysozyme, 11, 12, **17**, 19, 71, 73, 150, 153
  hen egg-white, 150

macrophage, 13, **14**, 17, 18, 19, 33, 34, 35, 37, 49, 70, 74, 120, 125, 126, 135, 148, Plates 2.1 and 2.2
  activation of helper T cells, 34, 35
  as an **antigen presenting cell** (APC), **33**, 37, 70
  possible role in self-tolerance, 120
  possible role in antigen-specific immunity, 125–6
  role in HIV infection, 135
  traffic through the body, 37
major histocompatibility complex (MHC), **31**, **60**, 61, 63, 115, 129, 132, 134, 138, 139, 140, 148
  see also MHC molecules, *H-2 complex* and *HLA complex*
Mak, T.W., 41
malaria, 74
malignant cell/transformation see cancers
Mantoux test, 143

marker molecule, **25**, 30, 31, 88, 106
mast cell, 13, **16**, 18, 19, 28, 29, 49, 52, 70, 71, 75, 102, 140, 141, Plate 2.3
measles, 72, 148, 153
Medawar, P., 118
membrane attack complex, **18**, 19, 28, 29
memory cell, **22**–3, 24, 28, 111, 113, 124, 135
   B cell, 24, 28, 111, 113, 154
   T cell, 24, 111, 124
MHC molecules, **31**–3, 41, 59, **60**, 78, 86, 109, 121, 155
   class I, 32, 33, **60**, 61, 63, 66–7, 86, 117, 129, 148, 155
   class II, 32, 33, **61**–2, 63, 67, 70, 117, 129, 139, 149
MHC restriction, **32**, 33
   see also self-MHC restriction
microbe, 5
microtitration plate, 99, 100
Milstein, C., 92, 94, 128
mitogen, 27, 108
molecular conformation, 8
monoclonal antibodies (Mabs), 40, **92**–4, 106, 108, 109, 110, 134, 137
   genetically engineered, 108
   human, 94, 108
   mouse or rat, 92–4, 108, 109
   production, 92–4
   use in cancer therapy, 108, 110
   use in leukocyte assays, 106
monocyte, 13, Plate 2.2b
monomer of an antibody, **48**, 49, 113
monovalent antigen or hapten, 76, 79, 81, 82, 90, 92, 95
morphogenesis, 88
mRNA
   effect of cyclosporin A, 134
   effect of interferon, 17
   RNA splicing, 56, 57, 58, 59, 113, 149
mucous membrane, 11, 12, 50
mucus, 11, 12, 50
multiple sclerosis, 139
multipotent stem cell, **12**, 36, 111, 133, 134
multivalent
   antibody, 90
   antigen, 76, 81, 82, 90, 92, 95
muscle endplate, 142
mutation, 58, 66, 72, 74, 121, 122, 145
   in breakdown of self-tolerance, 121, 122, 145
   in evolution, 72
   point mutation, 74
   somatic, 58, 66, 121
myasthenia gravis, 139, 142, 152, 158
Mycobacterium
   leprae, 74, 142, 143, 145
   tuberculosis, 74, 143
myeloma, 92, 138

N-acetylgalactosamine, 86
N- and C-termini of polypeptides, 42, 45
naive lymphocyte, **22**–3, 111

B cell, 22–3, 111, 112, 113
   T cell, 124
native (intact) antigen, 26, 84
natural killer (NK) activity, **15**, 16, 19
   see also NK cell
natural selection, 72
needle-stick injuries, 136
negative or positive feedback in the immune response, 18, 70, 123–4
Neisseria gonorrhoea, 73
neuroendocrine effects on immune response, 130–1
neurotransmitter, 13, 130
neutrophil, 12, 13, **14**, 49, 71, 125, Plates 2.1 and 5.1
nickel, 76, 143, 144
nitrocellulose paper, 104, 105, 157
NK cell, **15**, 16, 17, 19, 35, 71, 130, 136, 148, 153, 155
non-coding sequences of DNA, 55, 56, 57, 59
Northern blotting, 105
nucleotide sequencing, 43
nude mice, 137

oedema, 140
oligosaccharide antigen, 76
oncofoetal antigen, **137**
oncogene, **138**
oncogenic virus, 138
opportunistic infection, **6**, **133**, 135
   Pneumocystis carinii, 135
opsonin, **14**, 15, 16, 17, 19, 28, 29, 49, 111, 133
   acute phase proteins, 14, **17**, 19
   antibody, 14, 28, 29, 49, 154
   C3b, 18, 133
   in new-born, 111
opsonisation, **14**, 18, 19, 28, 29, 50, 153
organ-specific autoimmune diseases, 139, 145, 146
organ transplant, 134, 153
osmotic pressure effects in cytotoxicity, 16
Ouchterlony diffusion test, 96
Owen, R.D., 118
oxidising agents, 14, 15, 18, 74

pandemic, 74, 136
parasites,
   escape strategies, 74–5, 134
   immune response to, 9, 15, 17–18, 28, 30, 52, 71 74–5, 153
parasitic diseases, 5
   Chagas disease, 74
   filariasis,
   malaria, 74
   roundworm, 75
   schistosomiasis, 75, Plate 5.1
   tropical sores, 74
paratope, 25
   see also antigen binding site
passive protection, 50

pathogen, 5, 72
Pavlovian conditioning, 130
penicillin, 76, 85
pentamer of IgM, **50**, 87, 113, Plate 4.2
peptidoglycan, 17, 78
perforin, **15**
peripheral lymphoid system, **36**, 37
pernicious anaemia (autoimmune), 145
pigeon fancier's disease, 142
pH, 91, 97, 98
phagocyte, **7**, 14
   macrophage, 13, **14**, 17, 19, Plates 2.1 and 2.2
   neutrophil, 12, 13, **14**, 49, 71, Plates 2.1 and 5.1
phagocytosis, **7**, **14**, 18, 28, 29, 74
phylum, 6–7
physical and chemical barriers to infection, **11**–2
pituitary gland, 130, 131
placenta, 49, 50, 87, 111, 158
plaque, 108
   see also B cell plaque-forming assay
plasma, 16, 18, 36
plasma cell, **25**, 39, 52, 92, 108, 113, 154
plasmacytoma, 92
Plasmodium species, 74, 142
platelets, 12, 13, 49
Pneumocystis carinii, 135
pneumonia, 27, 111, 135
polyclonal activation of B cells, 27, 75, 134
polyclonal activator, **27**
polyclonal antiserum, 81, 90, **91**–2, 94, 95, 98
   production and purification, 90–2, 151, 156
   uses in assays, 94, 95, 98
polymers
   of antibody, 48, 49, 50, 51
   of antigen, 26, 27, 76, 155
polymorphonuclear neutrophil *see* neutrophil
polypeptide antigen, 8, 84
polysaccharide antigen, 17, 27, 76, 151
Porter, R., 41
positive or negative
   feedback, 18, 70, 123–4
   thymocyte selection, **117**, 157
pre-B cell, 112, 114
precipitation of soluble antigen, 90, 97, 98, 150, 156
precipitin reaction, **95**–8
   arc, line or ring, 96, 97, 98, 157
premature menopause (autoimmune), 145
pressure blotting, 104
primary adaptive response, **9**, 22–3, 27–8, 50, 59, 82, 124, 153, 154
primary and mature mRNA transcripts, 56, 57, 58, 59, 149
primary lymphoid organs, **36**, 37
primary structure
   of antibody, 25–6, 41–8
   of immunoglobulin superfamily, 67–8

of MHC molecules, 60–2
of T cell antigen receptor, 65–6
private idiotope, 126, 127, 134, 158
processed antigen, 33, 47, 84, 85
protease, 73, 140
protein A, 100, 102, 106
protein
    antigen, 76–9
    sequencing, 40, 43, 44
protozoa, 5
Pseudomonas aeruginosa, 73
psychoneuroimmunology, 131
public idiotope, 126, 127
purification
    of antibody mixtures, 91
    of antigen mixtures, 94–5

rabies, 72
radial immunodiffusion assay (RID), 96–7, 151, 156–7
radioactive labelling methods, 90, 100, 103, 105, 108, 109
    in cancer diagnosis or therapy, 108, 109, 137
    in **immunoblotting, 105**
    in **immunohistochemistry, 106**
    radioallergosorbent test (RAST), 102
    radioimmunoassay (RIA), 101–2, 103
    radioimmunosorbent test (RIST), 102
receptors
    for antibody Fc regions, 15, 16, 28, 29, 31
    for antigen, 20–1, **25,** 26, **31,** 41, 50, 65–6, 106, 112–3
    for EB virus, 31
    for interleukin-2, 124–5
    for opsonins, 14
    for sheep red blood cells, 98, 99, 107, 111, 114
receptor
    density, 124–5, 129
    library, 10, 78
red cell, 12, 13, 98, 99, 107
Reinherz, E., 41
retrovirus, 134, 137
reverse transcriptase, 134
Rhesus antigen (Rh), 86, 87
rheumatoid arthritis, 139, 146, 147
Rickettsia species, 74
    fevers, 74
RNA splicing, 56, 57, 58, 59, 113
rocket immunoelectrophoresis, 98
Roitt, I., 14
rosette *see* T cell rosette assay
roundworm infestation, 75
routes of infection
    general, 11
    HIV, 136

sandwich methods *see* immunolabelling
Schistosoma species, 75

mansonii, Plate 5.1
schistosomiasis, 75, Plate 5.1
second antibodies, 100, 102, 156
    see also anti-immunoglobulin antibodies
secondary adaptive response, 9, 22–3, 27–8, 48, 59, 124, 153
secretory piece, 50
self-epitope, 118, 119, 128, 139, 142, 145
self-MHC restriction, 115–7, 149, 151, 154, 157
self-reactive lymphocytes,
    B cell, 118, 119, 120, 121, 122, 145, 158
    mutant, 121, 122
    T cell, 118, 120, 121, 145
self-tolerance, 9, 51, 86, **118**–20, 121–2, 128
    breakdown, 121–2
    in idiotype networks, 128
    models of, 118–20
serum sickness, 142
sheep red blood cells, 98, 99, 107, 111, 114
sIg *see* surface immunoglobulin
signal transduction, 31, 65, 66, 67
size of antigens, 45–6, 76
sleeping sickness, 74
small lymphocyte, 12, 20, Plates 3.1 and 3.2
    see also B cell and T cell
smallpox, 83, 153
sodium dodecyl sulphate (SDS), 104, 105, 157
somatic cell, 52, 53, 55
somatic mutation, 58, 66, 121
somatic recombination, 55–9, 66, 112, 149
Southern blotting, 105
Southern, E., 104
spectrophotometer, 95
sperm whale myoglobin, 77
spina bifida, 98
spleen, 12, 36, 37
Staphylococcus species, 73, 100
    aureus, 100
Streptococcus species, 27, 49, 73, 111
    pneumoniae, 27, 111, 149, 154
stress and immune responsiveness, 131
structural domains
    in antibodies, 43, 49
    in immunoglobulin superfamily, 67
    in MHC molecules, 60, 61, 62
    in T cell antigen receptor, 65
suppressor factors, 34–5, 125–6
    see also lymphokines
suppressor T cell, 30, 34, 35, 75, 118, 119, 120, 121, 122, 125, 126, 128, 135
surface epitope, 76, 77
surface immunoglobulin (sIg), 25–6, 31, 50, 58, 76, 106, 112–3
surface marker *see* marker molecule
syngeneic strain, 64, 149, 155
synovial cell, 146
systemic lupus erythematosus (SLE) 139, 146, Plate 10.2

T cell, 8, 23–4, 30–5, 111
    antigen receptor, 31, 41, **65**–6, 106, 117
    cytotoxic, 30, 60, 66, 67, 71, 114, 125, 129, 135, 136
    delayed hypersensitivity, 30, 142, 143
    epitopes, 76, 77, **84**–5
    helper, 30–1, 33–5, 62, 66–7, 107, 114, 124–8, 130–1, 135, 142–3
    lymphokines, 34–5, 154
    rosette assay, 107
    self-reactive, 118, 120, 121, 145
    subset differentiation, 114, 115
    subsets, 30, 106, 107, 114, 115, 151, 158
    suppressor, 30, 34, 35, 75, 118, 119, 120, 121, 122, 125, 126, 128, 135
T cell-dependent antigen, 26, 27, 153
T cell-independent antigen, 26, 27, 75, 76, 153
T lymphocyte, 8, 23
    see also T cell
T suppression model of self-tolerance, 118, **119,** 120
TcR, **65,** 117–18, 155
    chains (α, β, γ, δ), 65, 117–18
    genes (*V, D, J* and *C*), 66, 117, 138
tertiary structure *see* higher-order structure
therapeutic uses of antibodies, 108, 109, 110
Third World diseases, 5, 6, 74, 75, 136, 153
Thy-1, 67, 68, 130
thymic epithelial cell, 114, 115, 117
thymic hormones, 117
thymocyte, 114, 115, 117, 157
    positive or **negative selection, 117,** 157
thymus, 24, 36, 37, 114, 115, 116, 120, 137, 150, 155
    Di George syndrome, 150, 155
    grafting, 116
    nude mice, 137
    role in self-tolerance, 120
thyroglobulin, 146
thyroid stimulating hormone (TSH), 146, 158
thyrotoxicosis, 139, 146, 152, 158
tissue culture, 92
    typing, 64
tissue-specific antigen, 87–**88,** 145
Tla complex, 63, 64
Tonegawa, S., 41, 52, 53
tonsils, 12, 36, 37
toxins
    bacterial, 29, 151
    in cancer therapy, 108
    lymphotoxins, 35
    lysosomal, 14, 28
traffic of leukocytes through the body, 36–9, 154
transfusion reaction, 86–7, 150–1, 156
transmembrane heterodimer, 60
transplant rejection *see* graft rejection
transplantation antigen, 60, 86, 109
tropical sores, 74

Trypanosoma species, 74, 75, 142
tuberculin hypersensitivity, 143
tuberculosis, 74
tumour-specific antigen, 108, 109, 137
two-colour cytofluorography, 106

universal donor, 87
upstream and downstream sequences in
  DNA, 56, 57, 58

vaccination, 5, 9, 22, 83, 153
vaccine, 5, 9, 74, 135, 136, 142, 152, 155,
  158
valency
  of an antibody, **48**, 49, 50, 51, 90,
  113–14, 149, 155
  of an antigen, 76, 79, 81, 82, 90, 92, 95
variable recombination, 57–8

variable
  domain, 44, 45, 65, 68
  region, 43–4, 45, 46, 47, 49, 50, 51, 54
  region genes (*V, D, J*), 54, 55, 56, 57,
  58, 59
vascular system, 12, 37, 38, 39, 49, 123,
  124
  circulation of leukocytes, 37, 38
  concentration of antibody, 49, 124
  concentration of antigen, 123
  high endothelial venules, 37, 38,
  Plate 3.2
vasoconstriction or dilation, 141
VDJ cluster or combination, 55, 56, 57,
  58
vertebrate immune systems, 6–7
vesicle, 13 *see* granule
viruses
  common cold virus, 150, 155
  cross-reactivity of cowpox and
  smallpox viruses, 83, 153
  Epstein-Barr virus, 31

escape strategies, 74, 135–6
human immunodeficiency virus, 134–6
immune response to, 9, 15, 16, 17, 29,
  30, 71, 133, 135–6, 153
rubella (chickenpox), 148, 153, 157

Western blotting *see* immunoblotting
white cell *see* leukocyte
Wiley, D., 41
Wu, T.T., 44

X-chromosome linked congenital immune
  deficiency, 133
X-ray crystallography, 44, 60, 61, 62

xenogeneic antigen, 85, 87–8
yellow fever, 72

Zinkernagel, R., 115, 116, 148–9

ACKNOWLEDGEMENTS

The author gratefully acknowledges the valued contribution of academic colleagues who commented extensively on earlier drafts of all or part of this Book—in particular, Anna Furth, Colin Walker and Sarah Bullock from the Department of Biology at The Open University; Professor Norman Staines from the Department of Immunology at King's College, University of London; and Dr David Catty from the Department of Immunology, The University of Birmingham. The editor, Julia Powell, the graphic artist, Pam Owen, and the designer, Sian Lewis, have contributed greatly to the Book's educational value.

Grateful acknowledgement is made to the following sources for material used in this Book:

Figures

Figure 3.13 Niels Kaj Jerne, *The Immune System*, copyright © 1973 Scientific American, Inc. All rights reserved *Figure 4.5* M. Schiffler *et al.* 'Structure of a type of Bence-Jones protein', *Biochemistry*, vol. 12, copyright © 1973 American Chemical Society; *Figures 4.16(a) and (c)* *Nature*, vol. 329, pp. 508-509, copyright © 1987 Macmillan Magazines Ltd.; *Figures 4.16(c), 4.17, 4.19 and 4.21* *Annual Review of Immunology*, vol. 6, copyright © 1988 Annual Reviews Inc.; *Figure 6.1* E. J. Holborow and W. G. Reeves, *Immunology in Medicine*, 1977, Academic Press; *Figure 6.8* *Advanced Immunology*, 1977 (1st edn), courtesy of Male, Champion, Cooke and Gower Medical Publishing; *Figure 7.3(b) and 7.4* Dr Catty, Dept. of Immunology, The University of Birmingham Medical School; *Figures 7.5(b) and 7.10(b)*: Dr S. Bullock, Dept. of Biology, The Open University; *Figure 7.6* Dr. D. Catty and Mrs C. Raykundalia, Dept. of Immunology, The University of Birmingham Medical School; *Figure 7.9(c)* Mr A. Scholey, Dept. of Biology, The Open University; *Figure 7.11* Dr H. M. Smedley, Kent and Canterbury Hospital; *Figure 8.1* *Immunology*, 1985 (1st edn), courtesy of Roitt, Brostoff, Male and Gower Medical Publishing; *Figure 8.6* courtesy of Dr Ray Owen and Gower Medical Publishing; *Figure 8.7* I. Roitt, *Essential Immunology*, 1977 (3rd edn) reported 1979, Blackwell Scientific Publishers

Limited, courtesy of Professor L. Brent; *Figure 10.1* British Medical Associated Board of Science and Education; *Figure 10.3* D. R. Stanworth, *Immediate Hypersensitivity*, 1973, Elsevier Science Publishers BV, Biochemical Division; *Figure 10.7(a)* Dr R. E. Church; *Figure 10.7(b)* Dr D. J. Gawkrodger, Royal Hallamshire, Sheffield; *Figure 10.7(c)* courtesy of the Royal Infirmary, Sheffield; *Figure 10.8* C. J. Webb, London School of Hygiene and Tropical Medicine; *Figure 10.9* Dr G. Hughes, Royal Postgraduate Medical School, London University; *Figure 10.10* Maclean Hunter Ltd, Medical Division; *Figures Q3 and Q6* first appeared in *New Scientist*, London, the weekly review of science and technology, vol. II, 1961; *Figure Q4* *Immunology*, 1985 (1st edn), courtesy of Roitt, Brostoff, Male and Gower Medical Publishing.

Plates

Plate 2.1(b) Dr P. Lydyard, Dept. of Immunology, University College and Middlesex School of Medicine, London; *Plate 2.2* Drs S. Gordon and G. G. MacPherson, Sir William Dunn School of Pathology, University of Oxford; *Plate 2.3(a)* N. J. Bigley *et al.*, *Immunological Fundamentals*, 1981 (2nd edn), copyright © 1981 Year Book Medical Publishers, Inc., Chicago; *Plate 2.3(b)* Electromicrograph by Dr C. G. Cochrane, from J. Bellanti. *Immunology*, 1971, W. B. Saunders Publishing, Inc.; *Plate 3.1(a)* L. Pachman, *Blood*, vol. XXX, p. 691, 1967; *Plate 3.1(b)* I. Roitt, *Essential Immunology*, 1974 (2nd edn), Blackwell Scientific Publishers Ltd.; *Plate 3.2* Dr W. van Ewijk, Erasmus University, Rotterdam; *Plate 4.1* courtesy of R. Dourmashkin and Gower Medical Publishing; *Plate 4.2* A. Feinstein, 'The 3-D conformation of IgM and IgA globulin molecules', *Annals of the New York Academy of Sciences*, vol. 190, 1971; *Plate 5.1* Dr D. McLaren, National Institute for Medical Research, London and Gower Medical Publishing; *Plate 8.1* Miss V. Petts and Blackwell Scientific Publishers; *Plate 10.1* Dr F. Bottazzo, Dept. of Immunology, University College and Middlesex School of Medicine, London; *Plate 10.2* Slide Atlas of Rheumatology, Gower Medical Publishing.